The Poetry Pharmacy Forever

William Sieghart has had a long career in publishing and the arts. He established the Forward Prizes for Poetry in 1992 and founded National Poetry Day in 1994. He was awarded a CBE in the 2016 New Year Honours for services to public libraries. His Poetry Pharmacy began touring in 2014; since then, and particularly since the publications of the hugely beloved *The Poetry Pharmacy* (2017) and *The Poetry Pharmacy Returns* (2019), he has prescribed thousands of poems up and down the UK over hundreds of hours of in-person consultations.

WILLIAM SIEGHART

The Poetry Pharmacy Forever

---

*New Prescriptions to Soothe,
Revive and Inspire*

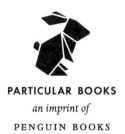

PARTICULAR BOOKS
an imprint of
PENGUIN BOOKS

PARTICULAR BOOKS

UK | USA | Canada | Ireland | Australia
India | New Zealand | South Africa

Particular Books is part of the Penguin Random House group of companies
whose addresses can be found at global.penguinrandomhouse.com.

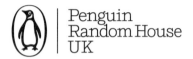

First published by Particular Books 2023
003

Editorial material and selection copyright © William Sieghart, 2023
The Acknowledgements on pp. 145–8 constitute an extension of this
copyright page

The moral rights of the authors and editor have been asserted

Set in 9.25/14pt Baskerville 10 Pro
Typeset by Jouve (UK), Milton Keynes
Printed and bound in Great Britain by Clays Ltd, Elcograf S.p.A.

The authorized representative in the EEA is Penguin Random House Ireland,
Morrison Chambers, 32 Nassau Street, Dublin D02 YH68

A CIP catalogue record for this book is available from the British Library

ISBN: 978-0-241-61128-9

www.greenpenguin.co.uk

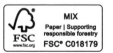

Penguin Random House is committed to a
sustainable future for our business, our readers
and our planet. This book is made from Forest
Stewardship Council® certified paper.

To Daniel Wolf

In memoriam

To Evie Prichard, my wonderful
collaborator in this project

To Donald Futers, who has edited the
trilogy, and to all my readers, who have
sent me so much inspiration

Contents

....

Coming Together

....

Moving Apart

Grief and Its Guises

Checking Out and Tuning In

Finding Light

Great Escapes

Introduction

In my introduction to the second volume of this pharmacy, I spoke of poetry's power as a spiritual link in isolating times. Little did I know, then, quite how isolating the times were soon to become. In the short handful of years since I wrote those words, the world has been paused and restarted, undone and remade. Isolation has been given a new significance, and the power of poetry to connect us has been tested in ways I never would have imagined.

As I write this we are all, I think, still reeling from the impact of the COVID-19 pandemic. Indeed, I feel confident in saying that as you read this, a year or even a decade from now, you too will still be carrying the psychological mark of those extraordinarily intense first months. Although most of us may now be settled and relatively safe in our 'new normal', there can be no underestimating the collective trauma of watching all our certainties dissolve, the loss of social connections and support structures, the fear of an unknown disease, and – for many – the death of loved ones on top of all of this. We are a society in greater need of comfort and compassion than ever.

During those first lockdowns, I was receiving daily emails from those who were struggling to cope with their new reality. People requested poems to salve their isolation, their grief and their uncertainty about the future. But most movingly of all, I heard from the health workers working in First World War conditions while we were locked up at home. They told me of their sense that they were living in a dystopian world entirely removed from the everyday lives of the rest of us. They went to wards full of death, every day, while we learned to bake bread and bashed our pans once a week. Despite all their training in dealing with the horrors that accompany the end of life, even they were unequipped to deal with the relentless devastation they were witnessing.

One incredibly moving message from a GP sticks with me. She had finally been released from her intense Covid rotation and returned to normal duties. And yet the world she discovered was far from normal. When she got back to her surgery, she found that two hundred of her regular patients had died since she had gone. *Two hundred.* 'How do I contend with this?' she asked me.

I am a poetry pharmacist, and so of course what I had to offer was poetry. And as the world became smaller and darker for so many of us, it was incredible to see the radiant and life-enlarging power that poetry took on. People were trapped in their homes, often alone or – maybe worse – feeling alone around those they loved the most. They lacked the words for the emotions they were feeling: the horror that seemed beyond expressing, the hope that felt too delicate to pin down. And so, they turned to others to say these things for them. The internet thrummed with poems shared, poems of comfort and recognition, old words that captured new circumstances with a burning precision.

It was during the first lockdown that I was approached by Emilia Clarke, of *Game of Thrones* fame. She had the wonderful idea of recruiting a fleet of talented actors to read poems from my pharmacy on Instagram, with my prescriptions written beneath. The reception from the public shocked all of us, and the clips took on a life of their own. By the end of the project we had donated thousands in royalties from the excess sales to her charity. Watching the poems I had once prescribed one-on-one in run-down libraries and literary festivals gain their own momentum, travelling across social media quite independently of me, and bringing comfort and joy to millions in the most hopeless of times – I can barely begin to describe how moving it was. The power of poetry, and of the public who shared it, left me awestruck.

If ever there was a time for transcendence, for poetry's power to transport and elevate, it was the years we have just weathered. If ever there was a time for human connection, poet to reader, through untold stretches of time and space to a common emotion, it was these fragmented and isolated months. And as we come to terms with what we have experienced, and with a world that has been forever changed, that complicity remains utterly essential. In the Introduction to the very first *Poetry Pharmacy*, I quoted Alan Bennett's description of finding the perfect poem 'as if a hand has come out and taken yours'. We have all needed a hand to hold recently.

Between the publication of the first and second volumes of this series, the Poetry Pharmacy took me all over the world. I prescribed poems across four continents, to people with every conceivable problem. Despite the fact that, this time, I have been forced to remain exactly where I was, I feel the pharmacy has travelled even further. Through the emails I've been sent, the posts and performances I've watched proliferate online, and the strange connections born of strange times, I truly feel that I have seen the power of the poems gathered by these books at work in the world, perhaps more than ever. Knowing that others took the same comfort in them that I did, through the same isolation: that has been the greatest connection I could wish for.

The History of the Poetry Pharmacy

I've always believed in the power of poetry to explain people to themselves. More than 20 years ago now, I used to flypost a poem around London at the height of the windows of a double decker bus. Called 'The Price' by Stuart Henson (and included in the first of these books), it's the kind of poem that has enormous impact and power, especially when encountered unexpectedly. I'd put it underneath bridges, where I knew buses would have to come to a halt at traffic. It was almost a guerilla tactic – confronting people with a poem that I knew would startle them. But I was also confident it could help them in some way.

Although I didn't think of it this way at the time, that may well have been the first incarnation of the Poetry Pharmacy. The Pharmacy proper began much later, while I was being interviewed at a literary festival in Cornwall, England, about a more traditional anthology I'd just brought out. A friend of mine, Jenny Dyson, had the lovely idea of allowing me to prescribe poems from that book to audience members after the talk. She set me up in a tent, with two armchairs and a prescription pad. It turned out to be all I needed. The hour we had originally planned for came and went, and then a second, and a third, until, many hours later, I was still in there, with queues of people still waiting for their appointments.

I realised that we were onto something. Suffering is the access point to poetry for a lot of people: that's when they open their ears, hearts and minds. Being there with the right words for someone in that moment – when something's happened, when they're in need – is a great comfort, and sometimes creates a love of poetry that can last a lifetime.

After Cornwall, I brought the Poetry Pharmacy to BBC Radio Four. I was asked back to do it again at Christmas – one of the most stressful times of year, as we all know – and then onto BBC television, and into the pages of the *Guardian* newspaper. Meanwhile, I never stopped doing my personal consultations. I toured the country, offering poetry pharmacies in libraries and festivals. In all of this, I learned how much most people's heartaches have in common. The objects and their circumstances might change, but there's nothing like listening to people's problems in leafy Kensington and then in a council estate in Liverpool for making you realise the basic spiritual sameness that runs throughout humanity.

I must have listened, over those first few years, to nearly a thousand people's problems. And then, in 2017, came the first *Poetry Pharmacy* book: a compilation of prescriptions that I had seen work time and time again, for the problems that really matter. Gratifyingly, readers took those poems to their hearts with just as much enthusiasm when encountering them on the page as they had in person. *The Poetry Pharmacy* became an astonishing success, and I found myself on the road more than ever before. Its successor, *The Poetry Pharmacy Returns*, followed quickly on its heels. And then, the world changed forever.

During the long months of lockdown, I felt the scope and focus of the *Poetry Pharmacy* shift, as my patients' needs and fears evolved. From that terrible time, I tried to retain the sense of perspective, of new priorities, that had blossomed from the wreckage of our old lives. Although in some senses this book is an ending – the third installation of a trilogy – it also felt like a fresh challenge, a new beginning.

And now, as I prepare to release this final volume of the series, I am struck by a miraculous sense of circularity. As I write these words, the first posters of my *Pharmacy* poems are beginning to be put up in hospitals, children's wards and doctors' waiting rooms across the country, ready to comfort those who need them most. The flyposting fanatic who pasted poetry under railway bridges has come full circle; a lot older, a little wiser, and just as passionate as ever. The *Poetry Pharmacy* trilogy may be complete, but I feel certain that its story is far from over.

How to Read a Poem

People are always telling me that they worry about their ability to read a poem. They don't really know how to. It's almost as though, when they're faced with a poem, they're instantly intimidated, even though of course they can read and write like the best of us.

When I'm asked for tips, I always give the same advice. Don't read the poem like you would a newspaper or a novel. Read it almost like a prayer. Say it aloud in your head as if you're speaking it to somebody else – somebody interested, who makes you want to perform it properly. Or, of course, read it truly out loud if you want to, and if you're not on the bus. Either way, it's the reading aloud that will allow you to properly hear it; that will make you understand the rhythms, cadences and musicality of the words and phrases.

When people tell me they don't understand poetry, I have another recommendation. I tell them to read the same poem night after night. Keep it by your bed, and read it before you switch off the lights. Read it five nights in a row, and you'll find you discover a totally new flavour and feeling from it every time. How you experience a poem depends on your own inner rhythms: what you've been through and what your mood is that day. But more than that, a really good poem is layered. It uncovers itself bit by bit by bit; never finished but always rewarding. That's why the joy of a really concise and brilliant poem is that you get more out of it every time.

Read the poems in this book however you like. Keep them in your desk drawer for when you feel shaky, or memorize them so you always have them to hand. Read them in the bath until the pages are crinkled beyond repair. But however this book works for you, remember that no poem deserves only a single visit. Come back, try again, approach it in a new frame of mind or with a new openness. If you persevere, you may be surprised at how many new friends you make.

Coming Together

Condition: Purposelessness

ALSO SUITABLE FOR: *disillusionment · failure · fear of mortality · skewed priorities · low self-esteem*

I found this little poem a particular comfort during the COVID-19 lockdowns. During those dark days, I, like many others, found a change of perspective pressed upon me rather unexpectedly. When my life was much busier and more complicated, full up with my various entertainments and obligations, it was easy to lose track of what was important. During the early days of the pandemic it was forcibly simplified, and I found myself welcoming my grown and almost-grown children back into a version of domesticity that none of us had ever really known together before. One small house by the sea, five people, a dog and no distractions. Suddenly, love truly was all that mattered.

It may not take a pandemic. It may be illness, old age or a conscious simplification of one's life – but eventually, each one of us will be forced to this realization. When life is reduced to the simple and all you can be is present to those around you, either physically or psychologically, the truth in the familiar wisdom becomes clear. Love – be it romantic love, love of family or love of friends – is what's important. Now, when I ponder my own mortality, my legacy and the value of my time on this earth, I do not count my material achievements and failures. Instead, I look to Raymond Carver, and his late wisdom.

It is not fame or success that warms us in our final moments. We do not weather lockdowns and convalescences buoyed by our reputations and our trophy cabinets (whether metaphorical or literal). Loving and being loved, knowing that you made life a more welcoming place for those you care about – this is what it all boils down to, in the end. The Beatles had it right all along – love really is all you need.

Late Fragment
by Raymond Carver

And did you get what
you wanted from this life, even so?
I did.
And what did you want?
To call myself beloved, to feel myself
beloved on the earth.

Condition: Need for Connection

ALSO SUITABLE FOR: *alienation from society • need for community • isolation • loneliness • social paranoia*

Lack of community is one of the great afflictions of modern life. For those of us in cities, it is possible to see more new faces in a half-hour on public transport than some of our ancestors saw in their entire lives. And yet what do we have to show for it? In that disorientating carousel of humanity, how many words have we exchanged? How many genuine connections have we made? It's little wonder so many people find themselves yearning for a romanticized picket-fence past, in which neighbours looked out for one another and front doors were left unlocked day and night.

Since its first publication a few years ago, I've been turning to this poem by Danusha Laméris whenever I feel that sense of disconnect creep up on me. For me and my patients, it's become a reminder that human connection is all around us, if only we know where to look. Laméris beautifully reframes the small banalities we exchange in public, finding in them the fellowship and generosity that, even now, can suffuse our relationships with the strangers around us.

We seem to be constantly bombarded with the message that the world is a dangerous place, and every unfamiliar face a new deceit; that we should stay home, board up our windows, and fade away – perhaps until those voices are the only ones talking to us. Thankfully, that is not the day-to-day experience most of us actually have. Instead, we give up our seats when needed. We pick up spilled shopping, or catch each other's eyes in shared regret when the train is delayed. We say 'bless you'. Every day, we build a world together, and it is a world built out of consideration and kindness and shared humanity. The language of grace resides in the simplest of gestures. It is our job to seek it out.

Small Kindnesses
by Danusha Laméris

I've been thinking about the way, when you walk
down a crowded aisle, people pull in their legs
to let you by. Or how strangers still say 'bless you'
when someone sneezes, a leftover
from the Bubonic plague. 'Don't die,' we are saying.
And sometimes, when you spill lemons
from your grocery bag, someone else will help you
pick them up. Mostly, we don't want to harm each other.
We want to be handed our cup of coffee hot,
and to say thank you to the person handing it. To smile
at them and for them to smile back. For the waitress
to call us honey when she sets down the bowl of clam chowder,
and for the driver in the red pick-up truck to let us pass.
We have so little of each other, now. So far
from tribe and fire. Only these brief moments of exchange.
What if they are the true dwelling of the holy, these
fleeting temples we make together when we say, 'Here,
have my seat,' 'Go ahead—you first,' 'I like your hat.'

Condition: Insularity

This very moving poem, used as code in agent Violette Szabo's reports back to Britain from Nazi-occupied France, is as inspiring a call to self-sacrifice as anything I've ever read. It reminds us, forcefully and beautifully, that our lives are never wholly our own. We live in families and communities: networks of love, duty and care that make demands of us in exact proportion to the nourishment they offer. The capacity to love broadly, beyond just ourselves and our own ends, is perhaps the greatest of all those that make us human; and as Leo Marks recognizes, it is most fundamentally a capacity for giving.

Often, when I talk to people about their troubles and worries, it strikes me that they would be vastly better served by devoting some part of their attention to the troubles of others instead. We have all had the experience of becoming trapped in the whirlpool of our own thoughts and desires, our own petty concerns and pride, until we have no sense of proportion left. Our pain and longing then seem all that matters, and everyone around us mere window-dressing. Yet this is a fantasy. When we look outwards, with empathy and care – when we allow others' needs to take on an equal urgency to our own – *then* we can at last begin to rationalize our feelings, and to recover a sense of scale. More simply, too, helping other people just feels good.

This is a poem about our capacity for love, and how far it goes beyond the romantic. It is about abstract love, the love we can have for those we have never met, and perhaps never will meet, and yet which is no less intense for its broadness. If we can tap into this love – which is really a love for humanity over the individual human – then no revolution, no sacrifice, should be beyond us.

The Life that I Have
by Leo Marks

The life that I have
Is all that I have
And the life that I have
Is yours

The love that I have
Of the life that I have
Is yours and yours and yours.

A sleep I shall have
A rest I shall have
Yet death will be but a pause

For the peace of my years
In the long green grass
Will be yours and yours and yours.

Condition: Rushing Love

ALSO SUITABLE FOR: *impatience in relationships · infatuation · first love · failure to live in the moment · romantic obsession*

Whenever I read this poem, it brings me viscerally back to those relationships of my youth that I choked with my eagerness. Caught up in my own vision of what I wanted the relationship to be, and who I wanted to believe my partner was, I tried to rush through the early stages and get to the good stuff. I thought that moving more quickly would sweep my partner along with me, skipping out all the uncertainty and awkwardness of the early stages of love.

It took me a long time to learn that people move at different paces, and that love is the sort of thing that simply cannot be hurried. Like happiness, any attempt to snatch it from the air will only crush its wings. After all, when you push a relationship beyond its natural pace, you are also pushing your partner beyond theirs. And even outside the bedroom, nothing is less attractive than a person who doesn't seem to intuit your discomfort, or even much care about your consent. Although danger is attractive in the abstract, when it comes to healthy adult relationships, we should all be looking for someone who makes us feel safe – and should be *being* that person, too, for those we love.

This poem is a lyrical lesson in how not to rush life and love. When we try to hurry through our relationships, we are also speeding past all the best bits. For all that the stories would have it happening at first sight, falling in love can be torturously slow; but it is the sort of joyful torture that you remember for a lifetime. Truly knowing someone, inside out and without judgement, is a lifetime's story. Nothing could be less satisfying than trying to skip to the final scene.

Down by the Salley Gardens
by W. B. Yeats

Down by the salley gardens
   my love and I did meet;
She passed the salley gardens
   with little snow-white feet.
She bid me take love easy,
   as the leaves grow on the tree;
But I, being young and foolish,
   with her would not agree.

In a field by the river
   my love and I did stand,
And on my leaning shoulder
   she laid her snow-white hand.
She bid me take life easy,
   as the grass grows on the weirs;
But I was young and foolish,
   and now am full of tears.

Condition: Taking Love Too Seriously

ALSO SUITABLE FOR: *fear of losing love • infatuation • romantic obsession • loss of perspective*

When we are caught up in the high drama of love, in its twists, turns and dead ends, it is easy to lose sight of the ridiculousness of it all. Which of us would sign up, clear-eyed, for having our brain chemistry sent into turmoil, our judgement skewed, our sense of self-preservation voided – and all for the sake of another person, no different to unafflicted eyes from the thousands of others we brush up against daily? What rational person would wish this bizarre condition on themselves? What kind of species would base its every film, book and song on such a mess?

In this witty poem, Sheenagh Pugh evokes all the absurdities and deceptions of love, including the fear of losing it. Yet she also captures the endless consolation that there is to be found in love. It distils our kindness, dissolves away our self-obsession, fills otherwise meandering lives with purpose and joy. Once we have tasted love, none of us would wish to give it up merely for the sake of a touch more sanity. Even love's miseries – and there are many – turn out to be worth it in the end.

I had a very wise friend who would always say to me, when I called him up to recount yet another romantic drama, 'One day you'll laugh about this.' Generally speaking, he was right. The gravity of relationships can be all-consuming when we are still in the thick of them, but sometimes all we really need is to take a step back and allow ourselves to laugh. Of all human activities, love is the least logical, the most fundamentally silly. And yet, somehow, though made from unlikely parts, it works – that's why Shakespeare's comedies always end in marriage. This poem is the chuckle we all need when we have begun to treat love like a tragedy, instead of like a comedy of our very own.

It's Only Love
by Sheenagh Pugh

It's just this judgement bypass, nothing drastic.
I'm told they do it without anaesthesia.

Leaves your conscience supple as elastic.
One of the side effects is mild amnesia,
Facts get reshaped, pain slips your mind.

Some blindness is normal,
Sufferers claim to see heaven on earth,
Stars in dull eyes,
Wit in unkindness.

This commonly resists all treatment given.
But it's not all bad.

Granted no flame retardant will work,
But the toxins are a tonic.

The virus leaves you selfless, brave and ardent.

Anyway, once you've got the thing it's chronic.

Most people learn to live with the condition.
What kills them is the terror of remission.

Condition: Growing Older in Love

ALSO SUITABLE FOR: *need for intimacy · choosing a life partner · maturing looks · loss of passion · loss of youth*

When patients come to my pharmacy bemoaning their lost youth and beauty, or the tremendous fun they no longer seem to have, I like to offer them this poem for a change of perspective. It is a reminder that growing old does not mean having to abandon humour, play or mischief – or, indeed, sex. Desire, like joy, does not depend upon youth and beauty. Often it flourishes best where there is profound connection, and long familiarity. If the years have also brought the odd smile line or love handle along with them, then all the better – these are signs of a life lived well, and in good company. When you really think about it, there is nothing more flattering than a smile line on a life partner's face.

I also like to prescribe this poem to those who are struggling to decide *who* exactly their life partner(s) should be. Bee Rawlinson alludes to a truth all too frequently overlooked in youth: that however beautiful we may be in our first bloom, physical beauty is never a solid foundation for a long relationship. Instead, it is the affection, the silliness and the sheer joy we take in one another that will bring lasting happiness and lasting desire. If you can't still fancy your partner in dentures and damp-proof smalls, then you're in for a rude shock in a few decades' time.

With the right person (or people) by your side, however, becoming older need not be something to fear or dread. Nobody can force you to be serious just because you are grey. In fact, the greyer we get, the harder it is for anyone to force us to do anything. We get to decide what our old age will be like – and although some might aspire to the bearing of an elder sage, there is nothing to prevent us from making our retirement a fabulously dirty comic romp instead.

Untitled
by Bee Rawlinson

Love me when I'm old and shocking
Peel off my elastic stockings
Swing me from the chandeliers
Let's be randy bad old dears

Push around my chromed Bath Chair
Let me tease your white nasal hair
Scaring children, swapping dentures
Let us have some great adventures

Take me to the Dogs and Bingo
Teach me how to speak the lingo
Bone my eels and bring me tea
Show me how it's meant to be

Take me to your special places
Watching all the puzzled faces
You in shorts and socks and sandals
Me with warts and huge love-handles

As the need for love enthrals
Wrestle with my damp-proof smalls
Make me laugh without constraint
Buy me chocolate body paint

~

Hold me safe throughout the night
When my hair has turned to white
Believe me when I say it's true
I've waited all my life for you

Condition: Lack of Passion

ALSO SUITABLE FOR: *need for physical intimacy • lack of excitement in love • longing for romance • losing the spark*

There's something wonderfully wholesome about this poem by Hugo Williams, so evocative of the marvellous complicity that arises when we walk about the world with a secret knowledge. That feeling of strolling down the road, grinning, and imagining that everyone can tell why it is we're so happy – that's a sensation that most of us have shared at one point or another.

Often, faced with an alienating world, we live our lives in our heads, and ignore or demote the importance of the physical and animal in ourselves. But what a shame that is. There is something transformative and life-enhancing about physical connection, which can often give us exactly the boost we need at the most unexpected of times. The wonderful lack of embarrassment and shame in the world Hugo Williams paints gives us a perfect blueprint for how we *could* treat sex: not as the insurmountable challenge, or trigger for bad memories, that for some of us it might guttingly have become, but as something we can embrace, an enriching and healthy part of life, and a joyful comfort in the darkest of times.

I love to prescribe this poem to those of my patients who fear that they will never again bump into passion in the grey streets of their lives. I see it as a reminder that sex, while being one of the most special things we as human animals share, is also nothing very special at all. Whatever Hollywood may imply, sex is not reserved for the most beautiful, accomplished or charismatic of the species. It is a great equalizer – a joy that transcends any of the divisions that undermine us.

However lonely or hopeless any of us may feel, it's important to remember that the opportunity for physical intimacy is never wholly fled. It may take some work, some confidence, a few bad dates – but for those of us who seek it, passion is always ultimately within reach.

Saturday Morning
by Hugo Williams

Everyone who made love the night before
was walking around with flashing red lights
on top of their heads – a white-haired old gentleman,
a red-faced schoolboy, a pregnant woman
who smiled at me from across the street
and gave a little secret shrug,
as if the flashing red light on her head
was a small price to pay for what she knew.

Condition: General Restlessness

ALSO SUITABLE FOR: *fear of commitment · boredom with the easy life · loss of perspective · discontent with stability*

From the outside, contentment is boring. So too is psychological stability. For anyone used to being tossed about on the currents of romantic anguish and interpersonal drama, the safe harbour of a calm life can look deathly dull – less a happy reprieve than a looming threat. And, true enough, as we age we very often complain that our lives no longer hold the buzz and excitement, the sheer sexiness and danger, that they once did.

So, is that chorus of our younger selves on to something when it tells us – echoed, perhaps, by the less attached, more risk-taking of our peers – that our lives of watching our gardens grow, of eating and sleeping and working, and being, essentially, our usual old selves, are all a bit boring? This poem by Wendy Cope has a wonderfully unexpected answer. Yes, it says: they are *utterly* boring – and that's exactly what's so brilliant about them.

The old adage holds that growing old is a privilege; I would argue that being boring is much the same. Indeed, the boredom that takes the place of past excitements is often the hard-won reward for all the work we've put into achieving stability, emotional balance and safety. Being boring is a trophy, symbolizing our evolution from thrill-seeker to mature adult.

When I find myself lamenting a slow period in my life, I remind myself that, whether as a result of tough external circumstance or, perhaps worse, of an insurmountable inner turbulence, not everyone gets the opportunity to be boring. It takes strength of character to embrace it, and a great deal of self-belief. But, whether we are ensconced in such stability now or living in fear of it, remembering how lucky we are can help us to see what a positive thing it really is. 'Being Boring' is my shortcut to that shift in perspective.

Being Boring
by Wendy Cope

'May you live in interesting times' – Chinese curse

If you ask me 'What's new?', I have nothing to say
Except that the garden is growing.
I had a slight cold but it's better today.
I'm content with the way things are going.
Yes, he is the same as he usually is,
Still eating and sleeping and snoring.
I get on with my work. He gets on with his.
I know this is all very boring.

There was drama enough in my turbulent past:
Tears and passion – I've used up a tankful.
No news is good news, and long may it last.
If nothing much happens, I'm thankful.
A happier cabbage you never did see,
My vegetable spirits are soaring.
If you're after excitement, steer well clear of me.
I want to go on being boring.

I don't go to parties. Well, what are they for,
If you don't need to find a new lover?
You drink and you listen and drink a bit more
And you take the next day to recover.
Someone to stay home with was all my desire
And, now that I've found a safe mooring,
I've just one ambition in life: I aspire
To go on and on being boring.

Condition: Need for Communication

ALSO SUITABLE FOR: *conflict avoidance · emotional repression*

One thing my pharmacy has taught me is that we can all recognize the anguish of things unsaid. There is no ache quite like that of lying next to the person closest to us in the world, and lying *to* them by omission the whole time; no dishonesty and discomfort quite like the pretence that everything is fine, when each of us knows that exactly the opposite is true. When we avoid difficult conversations in favour of that tense, alienating silence, we do a terrible disservice both to ourselves and to those we love. No surprise, then, that this sonnet – in the traditional form of a love poem – makes for a painful read.

Sometimes, when we fail to communicate a hard truth, it is out of cowardice. At other times, perhaps even most of the time, we do so out of a misplaced sense of kindness. But, as this poem so lyrically shows us, communication does not stop at language. When we cease to talk meaningfully with one another, we instead make our meaning clear through a thousand small gestures, touches and looks. What is unsaid is still sensed, still dreaded. We think we are saving our loved one from the pain of hearing whatever it is we are refusing to say, when in actuality all we are doing is adding weeks, months or even years of anxiety and paranoia to the eventual blow of the revelation. The pain is increased with every moment it is deferred.

One of our greatest blessings as human beings is our ability to speak to one another, to frame our deepest thoughts and desires in language and to find ourselves truly known by others as a result. When we turn away from that gift and try to cut ourselves adrift from those we love – that is when we are at our most unkind.

Repression
by Dorothy Nimmo

Something between them that must not be said
As if the words were fused and might explode.
There's small talk at the table and in bed
His body uses a mysterious code.

She reaches out again across the space
Between the things they mean and what they say,
He takes her clothes off but she hides her face,
He batters at the flesh he will betray.

So, without words they still communicate
And, close together, feel how far apart
They've come to be. Painfully celebrate
A broken contract somewhere at the heart.

It's growing louder, stronger every day,
The deafening noise of what they do not say.

Moving Apart

Condition: Claustrophobia in Relationships

ALSO SUITABLE FOR: *romantic indecision • falling out of love • feeling suffocated • need for gratitude*

At some point, most of us will find ourselves in a relationship so intimate, so cosy, that we feel smothered by it. Perhaps it has reached the point where we have to go out on our own just to feel ourselves again – which way, of course, temptation lies. In part, it seems simply to be human nature to long for the rush of instability whenever we find ourselves safe and supported; wonderful as it is to feel grounded by a relationship, that very grounding can leave us pining for the lurch in the belly we get when we look down from a great height.

These more destructive urges, willing us to choose danger and excitement over security and warmth, are the shadow side of a healthy relationship. And do you know? Sometimes that feeling might be exactly what we should be listening to. Sometimes we really have been bogged down by the wrong partner or the wrong life. Sometimes, taking a chance on change can bring a marvellous new direction to our lives, with all the new joys and experiences – and the new pain – that that entails.

But the thing to bear in mind, when we are weighing these choices, is just how much we tend to take for granted when we are settled and quietly content. The convenience and reliability of long habit can render the things we most depend upon invisible to us – and so blind us to just how amazing our partners really might be. How many of our lives' foundations are really built, not on our own strength, but on their love, attention and support? How many of our happy hours could, if we paused to think about it, actually be attributed to *their* levelling influence? This poem is a reminder, when you are chafing against the confines of a too-sheltering relationship, to consider what you have to lose, as well as what you have to gain.

Coat
by Vicki Feaver

Sometimes I have wanted
to throw you off
like a heavy coat.

Sometimes I have said
you would not let me
breathe or move.

But now that I am free
to choose light clothes
or none at all

I feel the cold
and all the time I think
how warm it used to be.

Condition: Breaking Another's Heart

ALSO SUITABLE FOR: *break-ups • letting go • self-recrimination*

We spend a lot of time dwelling on heartbreak, both privately and in the culture at large. Heartbreak is our great drama, the crux of innumerable books, films and midnight voicemails. What we fail to pay much attention to, though, is the peculiar pain and struggle of breaking someone else's heart.

Most of us see ourselves, at least generally speaking, as good people. Only the very worst of us derive pleasure from hurting one another's feelings. And yet a full and active romantic life brings with it, practically as an inevitability, the prospect of our causing agonizing pain to people who trust us implicitly. After all, there will always be times when feelings are not entirely mutual. Again and again, things will have to come to an end; usually, someone will have to be the person who ends them, and no matter how kindly and thoughtfully it is done, there is a good chance that the other person, hurt and disappointed, will resent them for it. More so than any other part of life, romance requires that we make monsters of ourselves, even if only in the eyes of our past partners.

This hurt is compounded by the feeling that we are not entitled to mourn the relationship we have ended – nor the self-image, specific to that relationship and that partner, that may have been shattered in the process. In this trenchant poem from Dorothy Parker, we are reminded of the importance of being gentle with those we discard, and mindful of others' hearts as we navigate our way through our relationships. But we are reminded, too, of the often unacknowledged pain of being the one who ended things – which, after all, sooner or later, all but the very luckiest and the very meekest of us will have to be.

A Very Short Song
by Dorothy Parker

Once, when I was young and true,
   Someone left me sad –
Broke my brittle heart in two;
   And that is very bad.

Love is for unlucky folk,
   Love is but a curse.
Once there was a heart I broke;
   And that, I think, is worse.

Condition: Siege Mentality

ALSO SUITABLE FOR: *lack of empathy • fear of the other*

I'm the child of a refugee, and I'm often reminded as I look at the news of the very plurality of the troubles refugees face. Not only do they have their own terrible stories to deal with, they have to contend with the hostility they all too often encounter in the country they arrive in, as well. Our media, our politicians: all seem to have a vested interest in stripping the humanity from those most in need of kindness.

This poem by Warsan Shire is a vivid and scarring reminder of the difficulties that many refugees have gone through in order to find a safe haven, wherever that may be. It cuts through the lazy portrayals of immigration that so often make cheap and easy headlines, but which utterly ignore the core facts of our shared human condition, and the real stories – the real lives – behind these most dangerous of journeys.

I've often said to patients at the pharmacy that one of the very easiest ways of dealing with our problems is to go out and help those whose struggles are far greater than our own. It's a sure-fire way to put our own private narratives of hard-done suffering into perspective, and to have brought home to us afresh the importance of looking deeper, thinking harder about what unites us, and being more accepting of otherness and difference.

It can be incredibly tempting when we encounter somebody who looks and sounds different to ourselves to see them as a threat, or at least as something utterly alien; and this is true whatever our skin colour, faith or background. When we do not make the effort to bridge that emotional gap, we deny ourselves the great gift of empathy; in preserving our own comfort, we cut ourselves off from the suffering of others, and, with it, from our own humanity. And with that, we lose whatever we might have thought we had to defend.

from *Home*
by Warsan Shire

No one leaves home unless home is the mouth
of a shark. You only run for the border when
you see the whole city running as well. The boy
you went to school with, who kissed you dizzy
behind the old tin factory, is holding a gun
bigger than his body. You only leave home
when home won't let you stay.

No one would leave home unless home chased
you. It's not something you ever thought about
doing, so when you did, you carried the anthem
under your breath, waiting until the airport
toilet to tear up the passport and swallow, each
mournful mouthful making it clear you would
not be going back.

No one puts their children in a boat, unless
the water is safer than the land. No one would
choose days and nights in the stomach of a
truck, unless the miles travelled meant something more than journey . . .

No one would leave home unless home chased
you to the shore. No one would leave home
until home is a voice in your ear saying – *leave,
run, now. I don't know what I've become.*

ALSO SUITABLE FOR: *need for forgiveness • guilt • regret • self-isolation • self-recrimination • shame*

In the wake of the global pandemic, a lot of people are feeling more alone than they ever have before. During the long periods of lockdown, many lost touch with community, old friends or colleagues. Even now that the world is beginning to reapproach a tenuous sort of normality, a sense remains that social muscles left to atrophy for so long may never return to their fullest strength; that loneliness is our new default condition in a world in which technology has rapidly taken the place of much normal communication and interaction. This poem is a marvellous reminder that there is always a welcome out there for all of us, however isolated or unlovable we may feel.

Humans are made for community, to love and be loved, and to brighten one another's lives with friendship. There are people out there who are perfectly suited to you, who are desperate to know you, and who would reach out if only they knew you wanted them to. Perhaps they are childhood friends; perhaps you have never met them before in your life. Either way, as long as you continue to stay inside, both literally and figuratively, they cannot welcome you. But if, as this lovely poem proposes, you go to them, you might be startled by the welcome you receive.

I also like to prescribe this poem to those who believe that they have transgressed unforgivably. They have broken promises, lashed out, harmed someone they love in a way they cannot reconcile with themselves. The shame they feel at their behaviour can keep them from reaching out and apologizing with the earnestness and generosity that might earn them forgiveness. But, as Rumi's poem knows, it is never too late, and nobody is ever truly beyond redemption. Suffused with kindness and inclusiveness, these lines reach out with the power of a warm hug from a stranger, to say: Come in. Stay a while.

Come, Come, Whoever You Are
by Rumi
translator unknown

Come, come, whoever you are.
Wanderer, worshipper, lover of leaving.
It doesn't matter.
Ours is not a caravan of despair.
Come, even if you have broken your vows
A thousand times.
Come, yet again, come, come.

Condition: Incompleteness without Romance

There is a terrible danger in expecting a partner to heal us. When we feel incomplete, inadequate, bitter and low, I think we've all been guilty of assuming that the love of another person will cure our ills. In pushing the responsibility for our wellbeing onto others, we are not just placing a terrible burden on them; we are also relinquishing our claim to be the master of our own inner world. How can we grow, mature and craft the tools we need to manage our sense of self-worth, if we have reneged on this most fundamental of duties to ourselves?

At first sight, this poem seems to be an amusing dismissal of any such responsibility. Dorothy Parker's list of symptoms might well be worthy of a brooding protagonist from Russian literature – but how serious can it really be, if it can be overcome by the simple expedient of falling in love? There is, however, a darker laughter to the poem, and its clue is in that final word: 'again'. The poem's speaker has been here before. Love has lifted her temporarily, distracted her – and then it has dropped her right back where she was, in the mire of her unhappiness. It isn't working. To try it again would be madness. Yet that is the toxic allure of the old familiar patterns.

The truth is that the incompleteness we all sometimes struggle with is not the lack of a person, or a possession, or a happily ever after. It is simply a reminder that we have work to do. If we delegate that work to someone else, we are doing everyone a disservice. And while it may be hard, it is also rewarding. It is cause for hope. This prescription is a redirection. You thought you needed love: go back to that list of contents, and think about what you're *really* grappling with. The first step on that road is the hardest.

Symptom Recital
by Dorothy Parker

I do not like my state of mind;
I'm bitter, querulous, unkind.
I hate my legs, I hate my hands,
I do not yearn for lovelier lands.
I dread the dawn's recurrent light;
I hate to go to bed at night.
I snoot at simple, earnest folk.
I cannot take the gentlest joke.
I find no peace in paint or type.
My world is but a lot of tripe.
I'm disillusioned, empty-breasted.
For what I think, I'd be arrested.
I am not sick, I am not well.
My quondam dreams are shot to hell.
My soul is crushed, my spirit sore;
I do not like me any more.
I cavil, quarrel, grumble, grouse.
I ponder on the narrow house.
I shudder at the thought of men . . .
I'm due to fall in love again.

Condition: Learning to Say No

Sometimes, the hardest word to say is no. Many of us are so conditioned to be kind, to be polite, to *take an interest*, that we find ourselves consenting to all sorts of social appointments and obligations that, given even an ounce more freedom to express ourselves, we would shudder at considering. So afraid are we that our dissent might hurt others, in fact, that we volunteer to allow ourselves to be hurt in their stead. Boredom, lost time, exhaustion, even burnout – how many are the forms of pain that we will inflict upon ourselves to shelter others from offence?

Whatever your upbringing may have taught you, your comfort and well-being do not matter less than those of the people around you. Your time is of no lesser value. Of course, it is good to be generous with others, to grant favours and extend a patient ear, but, crucially, only when you positively choose it. After all, you can't give freely what you've already exhausted; and greater still than your responsibility to humour those around you is the responsibility you bear to yourself. Fail in that, and you are letting down one of the very people who depend on you the most.

In this amusingly frank poem, Dennis O'Driscoll gives us a taste of what it might feel like to be honest, for once, about what we truly want, and to allow our true feelings, our true selves, to be seen by those who would take advantage of us. When I prescribe it to those who arrive at my pharmacy run-down and put-upon, I love to watch that sense of possibility unfurl within them. Yes, sometimes the most frightening word to say is 'no'. But sometimes it is also the most satisfying.

34

No, Thanks
by Dennis O'Driscoll

No, I don't want to drop over for a meal on my way
    home from work.
No, I'd much prefer you didn't feel obliged to honour
    me by crashing overnight.
No, I haven't the slightest curiosity about seeing how
    your attic conversion finally turned out.
No, I'm not the least bit interested to hear the low-down
    on your Florida holiday.
No way am I going to blow a Friday night's freedom
    just to round out numbers at your dinner table.
No, I'm simply not available for the excitement of your
    school-term coffee mornings.
No, strange though it may seem, your dream kitchen
    holds no fascination whatsoever for me.
No, there's nothing I'd like less than to get together
    at your product launch reception.
No, I regret I can't squeeze your brunch into my schedule –
    you'll be notified should an opening occur.
No, I don't appear to have received an invitation to your
    barbecue – it must have gone astray.
No, my cellphone was out of range, my email caught a virus,
    I had run out of notepads, parchment, discs, papyrus.
No, you can take No for an answer, without bothering
    your head to pop the question.
No, even Yes means No in my tongue, under my breath:
No, absolutely not, not a snowball's chance, not a hope.

Condition: Loneliness

ALSO SUITABLE FOR: *hopelessness • low self-esteem • self-isolation*

Life is full of calls to change. They can be disguised as discomfort, as sadness or boredom; but Warsan Shire's 'Today My Horoscope Read' zeroes in on perhaps the strongest of them all: loneliness. Short, memorable and blessedly simple, this is the kind of poem I love to find for my pharmacy: one that can be stuck to the bathroom mirror and used as motivation for the day, or, in this case, as the psychological kick in the pants we all need when we are feeling hopelessly cut off from the world.

Humans are social creatures at heart. Even at our most introverted, even when we *choose* to be alone, we still need to know that we are loved and accepted. Loneliness and perceived rejection, accordingly, are among the most painful stings we will ever know. Yet there is an extent to which even they are in the mind; and as with all thoughts that ail us, we can find ways to reframe them. As Shire says, we can become the alchemists of our loneliness.

We can do this in two ways. The first is to recognize the obstacles we have built to keep others out. Perhaps we have constructed walls of insecurity, telling ourselves that we are imposing on others when we seek their company; perhaps something else. The exact obstacles may vary – but they must all be torn down.

The next way of tackling loneliness is still more cunning: it is the splitting of *lonely* from *alone*. If we can only admit that not being around others does not necessarily mean that we are lonely, we can begin to take delight in our own company rather than dreading it – and to welcome our thoughts instead of batting them away. It's a strange alchemy. But there is an undeniable magic in the power we have over our own lives, if only we're willing to wield it.

Today My Horoscope Read
by Warsan Shire

You are the alchemist
of your loneliness.
You can create anything
in its place.

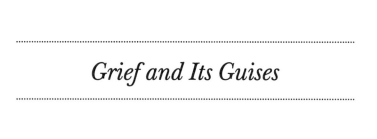

Grief and Its Guises

Condition: Unresolved Grief

When we mourn someone with whom we were particularly close, the hardest thing to reconcile can be the loss of the physical intimacy we used to share with them. Though the full intensity of their presence is lost to us, our need for it remains just as keen; and in our longing for a hug, a hand to hold, even just one last inhalation of their comforting scent, the sense of their absence is cruelly sharpened. That is why it can feel like such a miracle, almost a divine intervention, when we find them waiting for us in our dreams.

When we are granted that most unexpected of bonuses, the chance for a further encounter with a loved one, it is likely to be all the sweeter for the hours, weeks or even years that we have already spent grieving them. Details we thought we'd forgotten come back to us like precious gifts: the quirk of an eyebrow, a way of standing, a habitual phrase. Sometimes, even many years after their loss, when our memories are hazy and their face in our mind's eye has dimmed, we can receive a visitation and realize that they have lived fully formed in our subconscious all this time.

No; our dead never fully leave us, and when we dream of them – whether the dream is happy, painful or a blend of the two – it is also a marvellous confirmation that we have held onto their essence through all the travails of time and dwindling memory. They are branded into the very core of our psyche, never to be lost or dimmed. We discover that they have been with us all along, supporting us through our grief and our healing, even when we didn't know it; even when, consciously, we could no longer summon their image. What a relief that is, that nobody is ever truly lost to us.

The Embrace
by Mark Doty

You weren't well or really ill yet either;
just a little tired, your handsomeness
tinged by grief or anticipation, which brought
to your face a thoughtful, deepening grace.

I didn't for a moment doubt you were dead.
I knew that to be true still, even in the dream.
You'd been out – at work maybe? –
having a good day, almost energetic.

We seemed to be moving from some old house
where we'd lived, boxes everywhere, things
in disarray: that was the story of my dream,
but even asleep I was shocked out of the narrative

by your face, the physical fact of your face:
inches from mine, smooth-shaven, loving, alert.
Why so difficult, remembering the actual look
of you? Without a photograph, without strain?

So when I saw your unguarded, reliable face,
your unmistakable gaze opening all the warmth
and clarity of – warm brown tea – we held
each other for the time the dream allowed.

~

Bless you. You came back, so I could see you
once more, plainly, so I could rest against you
without thinking this happiness lessened anything,
without thinking you were alive again.

Condition: Grieving Differently

We've all heard that there is no right way to grieve, but it can be tempting to think that there are plenty of wrong ways. Human beings are hard-wired to forget the true intensity of pain once it has lifted, and from the outside, the pain of losing a loved one can be difficult to comprehend. At times, we watch people engaging in the most bizarre mourning behaviours, sometimes years after their loss, and simply find it baffling. These are sensible, intelligent people. Why, then, do they insist on making tea for their dead wife, or keeping rooms full of clothes that will never again be worn?

The truth is that grief is perhaps the most individual, and therefore the most lonely, of emotions. Even among families who are all mourning the same departure, each will have lost a different person within their own mind. This makes sense: when all of us contain multitudes, each relationship we have can hardly fail to draw out its own distinct version of our personality. Of *course* no one is ever lost to two people in the same way. How then, being so multiple in ourselves, so different even in our experiences of the same person, can we possibly expect to react identically to the temporary insanity of grief?

In this gut-wrenching poem, the speaker only begins to understand his father's peculiar ways of grieving when it is too late. Now, *he* is the one grieving strangely – and if he had seen earlier what he knows now, he might have saved his loved one from the doubled isolation of concealment and shame. This poem is a warning, a perfect example of how to make loss even harder. Its lesson is clear. The way we choose to grieve is valid – and so is everyone else's. Let's not make the darkest moments of our lives any more isolating than they already are.

Long Distance II
by Tony Harrison

Though my mother was already two years dead
Dad kept her slippers warming by the gas,
put hot water bottles her side of the bed
and still went to renew her transport pass.

You couldn't just drop in. You had to phone.
He'd put you off an hour to give him time
to clear away her things and look alone
as though his still raw love were such a crime.

He couldn't risk my blight of disbelief
though sure that very soon he'd hear her key
scrape in the rusted lock and end his grief.
He knew she'd just popped out to get the tea.

I believe life ends with death, and that is all.
You haven't both gone shopping; just the same,
in my new black leather phone book there's your name
and the disconnected number I still call.

Condition: Familial Loss

ALSO SUITABLE FOR: *bereavement · death of a loved one*

In times of grief, the sheer enormity of loss can be utterly overwhelming. The finality of it, that infinite list of never-agains that runs through the mind. We sit down with a familiar mug of tea, and reel at the thought that our beloved will never again sip from it; that that nonsense joke that once made us smile will never again be truly understood; that their particular way of walking down the stairs is gone from the world forever.

It is when my patients are struggling with this hugeness that I recommend they take a moment to contemplate this very calming poem – an extract from a sermon so powerful, so immediate and so timeless that it has long circulated in verse. In it, Henry Scott Holland speaks to us in utterly sensible and straightforward terms, just as I imagine my own dead would speak to me if they could.

Cutting through the emotional anguish of loss, we are reminded that our dead are never all that far from us. They can be pushed further, but only if we treat their memory as if it were itself dead, embalming it in solemnity and incense; only if we speak their name in hushed tones, and sever every connection we once had with the things we shared with them. But if we keep their memory alive with us, treating them with the same everyday love as we ever did . . . well, then, there they are, ready to answer us whenever we call.

The old life we shared has gone nowhere. Perhaps they are no longer physically present, but the structures they created together with us – the old jokes, the routines, all the building blocks of a life truly lived – those remain as long as we preserve them. They are who they were, and we, too, though we may have been changed by grief, remain fundamentally ourselves. Death is nothing at all. It does not count.

Death is Nothing at All
by Henry Scott Holland

Death is nothing at all.
It does not count.
I have only slipped away into the next room.
Nothing has happened.

Everything remains exactly as it was.
I am I, and you are you,
and the old life that we lived so fondly together is
     untouched, unchanged.
Whatever we were to each other, that we are still.

Call me by the old familiar name.
Speak of me in the easy way which you always used.
Put no difference into your tone.
Wear no forced air of solemnity or sorrow.

Laugh as we always laughed at the little jokes that
     we enjoyed together.
Play, smile, think of me, pray for me.
Let my name be ever the household word that it always was.
Let it be spoken without an effort, without the ghost of a
     shadow upon it.

Life means all that it ever meant.
It is the same as it ever was.
There is absolute and unbroken continuity.
What is this death but a negligible accident?

~

Why should I be out of mind because I am out of sight?
I am but waiting for you, for an interval,
somewhere very near,
just round the corner.

All is well.
Nothing is hurt; nothing is lost.
One brief moment and all will be as it was before.
How we shall laugh at the trouble of parting when
    we meet again!

Condition: Sudden Loss

ALSO SUITABLE FOR: *fear of loss* • *unexpected loss*

Sudden loss – loss for which we have had no time to brace or prepare – is a gutting experience. Between one heartbeat and the next, our world is unwritten and a new, emptier one takes its place. The white gate we knew on our strolls with a loved one may still stand in the field, the favourite park or the cherished street may still hold their usual place in our town, but they will never be walked through again with the same step, the same smile.

And yet, as Helen Farish brings home to us in this moving little poem, not knowing that the loss is coming can be something of a blessing. Instead of spending the precious final moments of those we love already in mourning for them, we can enjoy their company, unburdened by that terrible knowledge. Because the truth is, nobody can protect us from last times; but if we are lucky, we can at least avoid the burden and, in a sense, the contamination of knowing exactly when they will be. We can stretch those golden hours of safety and normalcy as far as they can possibly reach.

For this reason, I also turn to this poem in moments when I am most afraid of losing those I love. It reminds me that, although we cannot control how long we have with those we care about, we can control the quality of that time. Living in constant terror of losing what we have can, paradoxically, steal the joy of those moments still left to us. Better, surely, to surrender it all to God or to chance or to fate. Not to know, and not to wonder – simply to enjoy what we love while we can.

The White Gate
by Helen Farish

I'm so glad I didn't know
the last time was the last time
we went through the white gate
up the field, that I was able to turn
homeward happy. Lord, protect me

from last times and if you cannot
protect me from last times protect me
from knowing. Take everyone
suddenly, close the gate
suddenly. Tell me nothing.

Condition: Terminal Illness

ALSO SUITABLE FOR: *coming to terms with death*

It's an old piece of wisdom, but it's undeniably true: death puts our problems into perspective. Death can seem monumental, casting its shadow over everything, and never more so than when we know that it is coming soon, for us or for someone we love. Next to the enormity of life's ending, even the most all-consuming of our daily stresses soon seem to pale into insignificance.

There is no subject more difficult than mortality, and no situation more terrifying than a terminal diagnosis. In this marvellous poem by the late Helen Dunmore, however, the poet summons the most wonderful sense of beauty and calm out of that terrible moment. In doing so, she shows us something that is perhaps less obvious to those of us who have never crossed the Rubicon of such a diagnosis and reported back: that death changes our perspective in the other direction too.

This poem knows, you see, that small pleasures and simple joys can be magnified by their proximity to death, just as large problems can be diminished. It knows that the importance of living for living's own sake, of opening our petals and enjoying the bees' dance, is never more clear than when we are confronting its end. It is a crucial reminder that life can be lived in all its richness, right up until the final moment.

Receiving that most incomprehensible piece of news will never be easy. But if there is some comfort to be found, it is surely in this reminder that a life cut short can still be beautiful, and that an abrupt ending can still bring peace and resolution. We may not be able to choose when our finale comes, but we can always make the choice to keep flowering for as long as we can, drinking up the beauty and richness of experience until the last. Isn't that, in its own way, the most beautiful thing of all?

'My life's stem was cut'
by Helen Dunmore

My life's stem was cut,
But quickly, lovingly
I was lifted up,
I heard the rush of the tap
And I was set in water
In the blue vase, beautiful
In lip and curve,
And here I am
Opening one petal
As the tea cools.
I wait while the sun moves
And the bees finish their dancing,
I know I am dying
But why not keep flowering
As long as I can
From my cut stem?

Condition: Despair

ALSO SUITABLE FOR: *overwhelming grief · loss of pleasure in life · intractable misery*

It can be hard to imagine when we are out of love with the world, so choked by our grief and pain that it becomes a physical torture, that we will ever recover. Indeed, it can be hard to believe that anyone has *ever* felt this way and recovered. In the all-consuming grip of despair, it often feels easier to remain trapped there than to fight free.

Part of the reason I love this deeply evocative poem by Ellen Bass is that it recognizes the enormity of despair, and paints it so vividly that even those who are not struggling can feel its shadow in their bones. The suffocating weight of it; the incredulity that anyone could withstand this. Sometimes a poem does not comfort us in a conventional way, but instead offers us the gift of fellow feeling: the knowledge that others have faced the intolerable and survived.

More than this recognition, though, Bass also offers us a wonderful piece of advice about how to cope when our pain seems insurmountable. The thing, she tells us, is to love life. Not to love it for its pleasures, which in the bleakest times may be few and far between. No, instead we must learn to love life unconditionally, as one would an unruly child. We must love it despite, or even *for*, its horrors and miseries, just as much as for the joys and opportunities it brings.

This type of love, as anyone who has had their own love tested can tell you, is less a blessing than an act of will. Second by second, despite everything, we must choose to love life: to say to the world, as to a misbehaving child, 'You cannot stop me loving you. Nothing you can do will destroy my love for you.' It is only through this supreme act of forgiveness that we can begin to banish our despair, and discover how to live again.

The Thing Is
by Ellen Bass

to love life, to love it even
when you have no stomach for it
and everything you've held dear
crumbles like burnt paper in your hands,
your throat filled with the silt of it.
When grief sits with you, its tropical heat
thickening the air, heavy as water
more fit for gills than lungs;
when grief weights you down like your own flesh
only more of it, an obesity of grief,
you think, *How can a body withstand this?*
Then you hold life like a face
between your palms, a plain face,
no charming smile, no violet eyes,
and you say, yes, I will take you
I will love you, again.

Condition: Fear of Ageing

ALSO SUITABLE FOR: *need for humility • fear of vulnerability*

It seems to me that this extract, written when T. S. Eliot himself was no longer a young man, has a lot to teach us about what it means to grow old gracefully. Eliot lived in a society in which the elderly, especially old men, were treated with great reverence. Yet, as he himself approached that state, he recognized something fundamental about old age. We do not become intrinsically wise as we grow older; an abundance of experience does not necessarily yield an abundance of insight. What we do often become, however, is more proud.

Too little is said, I think, about the fear that is part and parcel of growing old. In our youth we feel invincible, immortal and unimpeachably strong. As we age, our fallibility confronts us in a thousand ways – in our face in the mirror, in our knees when we stand up, in our tiredness at the end of the day. Mortality is no longer a conceptual fear, but a tangible companion as we go about our lives. What Eliot understood about those old men, so feted for their wisdom, was that they were not dispensing disinterested insight, but reacting with defensive pomposity to their own fear of dying, or of losing their independence. In their fear, they resisted true connection, healthy change.

Instead of this reflexive self-aggrandizement, Eliot calls for humility. Humility, he says, is endless – and it is certainly true that for many of us, the times in our lives that have taught us the most are the ones in which we were humbled, or transported by a humble moment. Humility allows us to look at what we have lost without resentment, and to look ahead without terror or dread. Humility is the brother to vulnerability, which is the source of all human understanding and connection. That is what makes it truly wise. Wisdom should not set us apart; it should bring us together.

from *East Coker*
by T. S. Eliot

                    Do not let me hear
Of the wisdom of old men, but rather of their folly,
Their fear of fear and frenzy, their fear of possession,
Of belonging to another, or to others, or to God.
The only wisdom we can hope to acquire
Is the wisdom of humility: humility is endless.

Condition: Rage at the World

ALSO SUITABLE FOR: *despair at the absurdity of the world · grief*

When I was nursing my ailing mother in the last few weeks of her life, it struck me very clearly that although she was surrounded by family, as she withdrew and withdrew into herself she was very much alone. In the end, so are we all.

The cruel realities of this life tend to confront us when we are at our most vulnerable; when our hearts are at their most raw and sensitive. During the long hours at her sickbed, I had ample time to contemplate life's absurdities and unfairnesses. I was filled with a kind of directionless anger, not aimed at any individual, but instead at a world that demands such sacrifices of us; at a world that tells us that, in order to live, we must endure the loss of those we love, and sets as a prerequisite of life the terrible solitude of death. A world which would blithely continue to exist without my mother in it.

Throughout that vigil, I would often turn to this poem, and find within it the peace that would allow me to retain my equilibrium in that awful time. Through it I was reminded that although nature can be painful and lonely, it is not malicious. The clouds and the mountains do not know how to be cruel; they do not even know how to be beautiful. They simply are. It is we who reflect our emotions back upon them. The laws of the universe, of birth and death, are just the same. The immensity and indifference of the world may make it terrible, but they are also what make it beautiful. Once we have truly understood this we can surrender our anger, and learn to forgive the world for being as it must be.

High Country Weather
by James K. Baxter

Alone we are born
And die alone;
Yet see the red-gold cirrus
Over snow-mountain shine.

Upon the upland road
Ride easy, stranger:
Surrender to the sky
Your heart of anger.

Condition: Weathering Sorrow

ALSO SUITABLE FOR: *avoidance of pain · disconnectedness · emotional repression*

In the course of a life that has held many moments of joy and many moments of anguish, I find that I've learned the most through sorrow. More often than not, when everything is running smoothly, we are merely skating over the surface of our lives and of our selves. In times of trouble, when we feel ourselves submerged and struggling – that's when we plumb our own true depths.

Sorrow forces us to encounter the darkness in our souls. In doing so, it offers us the opportunity to acknowledge that darkness – to confront it. This takes reserves of strength and determination that, in the frictionlessness of our happier days, we may never have had cause to exercise. Yet, if we are open-hearted, it can also bring us to a new empathy and understanding for others that is almost invariably closed to those who have never known the depths. Strange as it may seem, there is a humility and a fellow feeling born of learning just how low one can go that seems to be all but impossible to attain in any other way.

Ultimately, life is not just about seeking pleasure and ease, and lounging about where we've found them like dragons on piles of gold. Being a human being is about evolution, self-knowledge and our connections with others, and it is through those periods in which we are hurt the most terribly that we are most able to cultivate our humanity. That, in the end, is what deepens us; that's what leaves us better equipped to help others, and what leaves others better equipped to help us in their turn. So the next time you are given a box of darkness, know it for what it is: a gift of depth, and a gift of growth.

The Uses of Sorrow
by Mary Oliver

(In my sleep I dreamed this poem)

Someone I loved once gave me
a box full of darkness.

It took me years to understand
that this, too, was a gift.

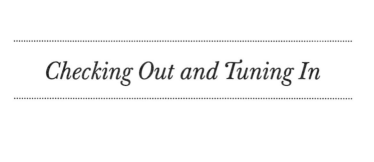

Checking Out and Tuning In

Condition: Stagnancy in Motion

ALSO SUITABLE FOR: *need for initiative · lack of spontaneity · loss of zest for life*

When we look back through the rear-view mirrors of our lives, it is tempting to mourn the stops we never made, and all those moments we were too fixated on the motorway to notice. We think of the people we never met, the opportunities we missed, the nights we never danced away because, we told ourselves, we knew where we were going: we had things to achieve, and we weren't going to accomplish them by pausing to experience the unplanned and unexpected.

Perhaps we worry we have been on autopilot, cruising past these opportunities without the initiative to press the brakes. Or perhaps, instead, we have been accelerating too hard: flooring the pedal and leaving what could have been our greatest adventures reeling in the dust.

The difficulty is that great things tend not to happen if we don't take at least some of the initiative needed to *make* them happen. When we are living in a frenetic blur, or a haze of cynicism, it is easy to dismiss the idea that there might be any good surprises left out there to discover. But this poem reminds us that that simply isn't the case. There is always something to be excited about, something that will return our excitement in equal measure. We must have the presence of mind, the willing, and, most of all, the optimism to help the moment meet us halfway.

Your greatest hour could be just around the corner, or just beyond the horizon. All it asks of you is that you reach out to it. So when you next sense an opportunity on the horizon, press the brakes. Open the door and leave the safe bubble of the car behind. You never know what beautiful thing might be waiting, breath held, for your arrival.

Horizon
by Rudy Francisco

I hope I haven't already driven
past my greatest moments.

I hope there is something
beautiful on the horizon
that's just as impatient as I am.
Something so eager,
it wants to meet me halfway.
A moment that is diligently
staring at its watch, trembling with
nervousness, frustrated,
and bursting at the seams,
wondering what's taking me
so long to arrive.

Condition: Need for Change

It can be comforting to imagine that it is external factors that drive the strife and struggle of life. All will be well, we tell ourselves, just as soon as we have that new job, the perfect partner and the colour coordinated pencil pots of our dreams. Yet, if we can summon the humility – and the bravery – to look honestly at ourselves, most of us will find that it is really our own patterns of behaviour and thinking that sit at the root of our troubles. Whether in our neuroses, our habits, our fears or our methods of deflecting them, the enemy, all too often, lies within.

I recognize this in myself, and I see it frequently in those patients who come to me complaining of anger with the world. All too often, the truth is that it's not circumstances we are raging against, but our own inability to change. We lack the courage to ask ourselves: 'Why am I still banging my head against the same wall?'

When I prescribe this concise and incisive poem, I don't do so to discourage people from changing the world. There are few of us, I think, who would not agree that it could benefit from change in all manner of ways. Rather, it is when we seek to change the world around us not for itself, but in order to achieve our *own* happiness or fulfilment, that we should turn to these lines.

Changing oneself for the better, even identifying the changes that need to be made, can be one of the hardest tasks of a lifetime. There's no shame in seeking help with it, whether from a trusted friend or a professional. But if we're prepared to do the hard work of facing up to our own flaws, we might be able to do the most important thing of all: to change ourselves. And in changing ourselves, we can change everything.

Yesterday I Was Clever
by Rumi
translator unknown

Yesterday I was clever, so I wanted to change the world.
Today I am wise, so I am changing myself.

Condition: Slowing Down

ALSO SUITABLE FOR: *insecurity about ageing*

Acknowledging the end of one's youthful vitality can be a very difficult adjustment – yet there comes a point at which it is simply impossible to keep up with the younger generation. Take me: even if I had the will or the interest to keep up with Gen Z's fashion and music, I know better than to deceive myself that they would want me to.

The sad thing, though, is that as we older folk lose our energy, we can often lose our confidence along with it. We may think that we've lost not only our youthfulness, but also our usefulness, our power to entertain and inspire. And if we are no longer the life and soul of the party, we ask ourselves, why should we be invited at all? Meanwhile, life's more visceral pleasures begin to dwindle. We are settled down, responsible, and acutely aware of the possibility of a three-day hangover.

That is where this charming poem by Roger McGough comes in, reminding us in wonderfully witty terms that it is never too late to be a little wild. Yes, perhaps our energies are dwindling. Perhaps we are at our happiest tucked in with a hot water bottle by the *Six O'Clock News*. But there are plenty of hours in the day, and, with a little creativity, it's possible to pack a staggering amount of excitement in before an early bedtime. There is no shame in slowing down; but there is a great deal of pride to be found in having fun on one's own terms.

Scintillate
by Roger McGough

I have outlived
my youthfulness
so a quiet life for me

where once
I used to
scintillate

now I sin
till ten
past three.

Condition: Time-wasting

ALSO SUITABLE FOR: *inertia • failure to live in the moment •
self-absorption • taking life for granted*

When this wonderful poem by Nâzım Hikmet tells us to live
seriously, it does not mean that we should live without humour
and play. In fact, quite the opposite. But what it does mean is
that we must not live *lightly*. We must not allow our lives to tick
away without notice, appreciation, joy in the very act of living.
We must be enthralled by the reality of it, the sheer improbable
wonder of being and staying alive, and doing all of those things
that make up an existence.

So many people come to talk to me about their sense of *what if*,
and the heavy weight of ambitions unrealized. They spend their
lives sitting and waiting and musing, thinking about what might
be, rather than actually just being. Here, Hikmet tells us that living
must be our whole occupation, and in this deft phrase he rules
out all the preoccupations that can keep us from living at all. Petty
worries, jealousies and distractions can blind us to the everyday
miracles all around us. Instead, he says, we should live like
squirrels – utterly absorbed in the process of *being*, instead of
looking for some notional narrative or attainment larger than it.

Of course, Hikmet does not only talk about squirrels. Above
all, this poem reminds us that we owe something to life itself.
We have an obligation to make use of every day, every hour, every
moment – even if by 'making use' we simply mean paying attention. And, though most of us will never find ourselves with our
hands tied and our backs to the wall, nor risking our lives in a
laboratory, what I've often counselled my patients remains true:
to put our energies to the service of others can be the ultimate
salve for the guilt of selfishness and waste. There is such inordin-
ate value in life itself; how can we possibly take it for granted?

from *On Living*

by Nâzım Hikmet

translated by Randy Blasing and Mutlu Konuk

Living is no laughing matter:
      you must live with great seriousness
            like a squirrel, for example –
  I mean without looking for something beyond and above living,
            I mean living must be your whole occupation.
Living is no laughing matter:
      you must take it seriously,
      so much so and to such a degree
  that, for example, your hands tied behind your back,
                your back to the wall,
  or else in a laboratory
      in your white coat and safety glasses,
      you can die for people –
  even for people whose faces you've never seen,
  even though you know living
      is the most real, the most beautiful thing.
I mean, you must take living so seriously
  that even at seventy, for example, you'll plant olive trees –
  and not for your children, either,
  but because although you fear death you don't believe it,
  because living, I mean, weighs heavier.

Condition: Fear of Pain

None of us will manage to live a life free from pain. As a parent, this can be an especially difficult truth to accept. Disappointment, grief, hurt feelings: all of these are an integral part of any human life. Indeed, it has often been argued that pain is so intricately bound up with its opposite extreme, joy, as well as with love, that a life without one would necessarily be a life without the others, too. Given that, which of us would wish upon anyone a life without the opportunity for pain?

Then again, if we cannot protect ourselves and our loved ones from pain, what *are* we to do with it? How can we reconcile ourselves to the certainty of future agony? The answer lies in these wise words by Teddy Macker, which make plain the essentially transformative power of pain. Pain is a part of things, he tells us. It is as natural as breathing, and just as essential to life. We are stretched and changed by pain in ways that can carry us through into gentler seasons, stronger, wiser and richer with fertile possibility than we were before we were challenged. And once we have reached that greater maturity, we will look back on those painful periods and be proud of our own resilience, our own capacity for feeling.

Macker's most crucial insight is that it takes effort to realize pain's potential. For every story of a person transformed by their pain, we can find someone who was calcified by it instead, or sought to avoid it with drink or drugs. Like compost, our troubles need to be turned, known and honoured if they are to become the rich, fruitful soil in which we can grow. It is our responsibility not to flinch from pain, but to process it and learn from it. If we can make that effort, then pain need never be our enemy again.

from *Poem for My Daughter*
by Teddy Macker

It seems we have made pain
some kind of mistake,
like having it
is somehow wrong.

Don't let them fool you –
pain is a part of things.

But remember, dear Ellie,
the compost down in the field:
if the rank and dank and dark
are handled well, not merely discarded,
but turned and known and honored,
they one day come to beds of rich earth
home even to the most delicate rose.

Condition: Need for Bravery

ALSO SUITABLE FOR: *fear • fragility • need for guidance • need for reassurance*

When we are feeling frightened or small or fragile, doubting our own power to overcome the hurdles we face, we tend to look to external forces for rescue. If we are religious, perhaps we pray for help, or for deliverance from hardship. If we are secular, we may turn to any number of strategies, from seeking someone else to shoulder our burden, to just sticking our heads in the sand and hoping it will all go away.

In this poem, Rabindranath Tagore understands that there is a lot to be said for looking within, instead of without, when we are at our lowest points. For me, his lines are a reminder that whatever higher forces we may believe in, whether spiritual or earthly, we can find and amplify their echo within ourselves. By holding to our own courage, love and strength, we can become a reflection of the very thing that we are asking to save us.

For Tagore, that meant God. For others, it may be grace, community or a sense of humanity's collective capacity to overcome. Whatever that external force may be for you, in your humility before it you can find strength, and a reassuring voice that tells you that you have the patience, and the endurance, to overcome.

Tagore's poem has one final message: that not only our successes, but our failures, too, are gifts. Marvellous as success feels, it offers us little opportunity to evolve, nor to strengthen the muscles that allow us to keep fighting. Only through our hardships can we learn to become the person *we* have needed at our own lowest points – and to be that person not just for ourselves, but for others, too. In the process, we might give those around us an even greater gift: the example of courage and acceptance. That's something we can all aspire to, no matter our system of beliefs.

Let Me not Pray
by Rabindranath Tagore

Let me not pray to be sheltered from dangers
but to be fearless in facing them.

Let me not beg for the stilling of my pain
but for the heart to conquer it.

Let me not look for allies in life's battlefield
but to my own strength.

Let me not crave in anxious fear to be saved
but hope for the patience to win my freedom.

Grant that I may not be a coward,
feeling Your mercy in my success alone;

But let me find the grasp of Your hand in my failure.

Condition: Need to Take Control

ALSO SUITABLE FOR: *need for fire in the belly • feelings of powerlessness*

Written over 140 years ago, William Ernest Henley's 'Invictus' is one of those poems from a different era that has been sent to me so many times, by so many readers, that it's clear something about it continues to speak to us across the centuries. There is something heroic in the way it describes overcoming the challenges of life by taking responsibility for and control over one's own path. It makes no attempt to diminish life's struggles, the maelstrom of chance and loss and fear that many of us battle against during the hardest times. It acknowledges our pain and dread. And yet it also brings hope that we can surmount our troubles, no matter what they may be.

The key to this poem is in its final two lines, written with such conviction and driving rhythm that they could be a mantra to march through life to. Henley tells us that we are the masters of our fate, and that therefore everything is endurable. While we direct our own lives, set our own course and choose our battles, we can never be overwhelmed. However difficult things may become, we will know that we didn't allow ourselves to be swept away by fate, but instead chose to steer through the storm, driven by our faith that we could weather it.

Nowadays, technology allows for unprecedented intrusions into our lives, in a world governed by algorithms beyond our comprehension. It can be easy to assume that the course of our lives is beyond our control; that there are forces greater than us which determine our direction, and even our ability to overcome. Even now, however, this poem reaches out to bring home to us the fundamental indomitability of the human spirit. Our free will is our greatest defence and hope against any difficulty. We govern our lives. We own our futures. We are the captains of our souls.

Invictus
by William Ernest Henley

Out of the night that covers me,
　　Black as the pit from pole to pole,
I thank whatever gods may be
　　For my unconquerable soul.

In the fell clutch of circumstance
　　I have not winced nor cried aloud.
Under the bludgeonings of chance
　　My head is bloody, but unbowed.

Beyond this place of wrath and tears
　　Looms but the Horror of the shade,
And yet the menace of the years
　　Finds and shall find me unafraid.

It matters not how strait the gate,
　　How charged with punishments the scroll,
I am the master of my fate,
　　I am the captain of my soul.

Condition: Choosing a Life

ALSO SUITABLE FOR: *indecision • regret • second-guessing • speculating about the past • what ifs*

Once we've reached a certain age, very few of us can truly claim to have no regrets; we all have our share of *what ifs* and *if onlys*, and as we grow older, taking more and more consequential decisions, their numbers only swell. Very often, it is these niggling regrets that drive patients to my pharmacy. What if I'd married the other suitor, they ask; what if I'd taken the other job; what if I'd moved to the faraway city – or, on the contrary, stayed put? Worked harder? Taken more time with family? Had children? Stayed single? When we are dissatisfied, it is tempting to dwell on those wonderful other lives that we convince ourselves could have been.

Linda Pastan's 'Commencement Address' reminds us that no choice is clear, and no path leads to unadulterated happiness. Whatever life we choose to pursue, it will bring with it its own disappointments and frustrations. Wealth comes and goes, often for reasons we could never have predicted. So much of life is chance, and so much of every choice is unknowable. Perhaps this sounds nihilistic, but it is also a fantastic relief. What is the point of flagellating ourselves for taking the wrong path, if we cannot know that any other would have been smoother? Perhaps, in the end, none of our choices is ever *truly* transformative. Perhaps we are both the wise man and the fool, and must learn to love both equally.

Somehow, through this disillusionment, we reach a greater meaning. As Pastan shows us at the end of the poem, our choices and our regrets are not really what matter. The sun and the moon, the blood in our veins, the water that soothes us, the air we breathe – if we attend to what is really around us, we will see that wasting time on *what ifs* is the most foolish thing of all.

Commencement Address
by Linda Pastan

If you live on the cutting edge,
surely you'll get cut.

If you live the simple life,
it won't be simple.

If you sit at a desk composing words
the alphabet will mock you,

or you'll drown in the currents
of the page.

Work hard. Be lazy.
Money will come and go

like green leaves in their season.
But don't forget

the wise man and the fool
are blood brothers.

At the end
what matters

is the sun, the moon:
arterial red, bone white.

Condition: Need for Healing

ALSO SUITABLE FOR: *despair · heartbreak · impatience in recovery · need for self-care · struggling to cope*

When the blows of life are raining down, when we are overcome by miseries and reeling with pain, often what we need most of all is the simple permission to curl up and protect ourselves as best we can. Sometimes, in the thick of adversity, it is just not the time to hurl yourself out into the big wide world and try to turn things around. It is enough of a struggle just to endure, to remain whole, and to live to fight another day.

Though first published as part of a longer poem written for a break-up, these lines have come to speak to readers about much more than just heartbreak. Whatever your troubles or misfortunes, they are a reminder of the importance of being respectful of your own vulnerabilities, and of recognizing the strength and resolve it takes to be kind when it feels like no one and nothing else in the world is doing the same. As John O'Donohue so movingly puts it, 'If you remain generous, / Time will come good.' Even at the best of times, generosity is not always an easy virtue to practise; but generosity towards yourself, whether that means a kind word or even permission to cry, can be fantastically difficult to summon when your every instinct is to self-flagellate instead.

The truth of the matter is that it's not when we're in the midst of the storm that we should stand and fight. That is the time to shelter, to lie low, to hold on to our sense of ourselves and to carve out what space we can in a hostile world. The time to process the pain, on the other hand – to inspect and analyse and rebuild – comes after the cruel weather has passed. Until then, the important thing is to be generous. Give yourself the gift of patience, and wait for the sunnier days when you will embark on the new beginning of recovery.

'This is the time to be slow'
by John O'Donohue
Excerpt from *A Blessing for the Break-up of a Relationship*

This is the time to be slow,
Lie low to the wall
Until the bitter weather passes.

Try, as best you can, not to let
The wire brush of doubt
Scrape from your heart
All sense of yourself
And your hesitant light.

If you remain generous,
Time will come good;
And you will find your feet
Again on fresh pastures of promise,
Where the air will be kind
And blushed with beginning.

ALSO SUITABLE FOR: *disconnectedness • loneliness*

I am regularly astounded by the degree of self-absorption that it takes just to survive in this world we've built. In the major cities, we live jostled by thousands of people a day whose lives are just as rich and fraught and emotionally intense as our own. The man making our morning coffee, the woman who treads on our foot on the bus, the busker playing for change on the street corner: each of their worlds is an intricate, many-layered tapestry, just as mysterious and vivid as your own. And if any of us allowed ourselves truly to recognize this, to reckon with everything it entails, day in and day out – well, how would we ever get anything done?

Challenging as it is, finding space to integrate this knowledge into our lives is also vitally important. So often in our busy, frenetic world, we can lose track of the fundamental humanity of those around us. People can come to seem reduced to their function, so that we might as well be navigating a world populated by movie extras, with no character motivation beyond their significance to the central plot (by which, of course, I mean our own, endlessly fascinating lives).

The truth is that each human mind is a universe of its own – and a part of the universe (or, as the Persian poet Hafez puts it, God) speaking. Every person we meet and dismiss, whether through prejudice or simply because we do not have time to engage with them, has something valuable to contribute; and our lives, however endlessly fascinating they may be, can only be enriched by making space for the humanity of those we find around us. Provided we learn how to truly listen, we need never be bored or lonely again.

Everyone is God Speaking
by Hafez
translator unknown

Everyone is God speaking.
Why not be polite and listen to Him?

Condition: News Addiction

ALSO SUITABLE FOR: *anxiety · doomscrolling · emotional self-sabotage*

Digital addiction can take all kinds of forms. Some may push themselves to their limits to achieve the next flurry of 'likes'; some bankrupt themselves in online games. Like many people, my rather more mundane form of addiction is to rolling news. Newspaper apps, news alerts, Twitter: these days there is a whole banquet of disaster open to us at the flick of a finger.

Endless scrolling can seem rather more virtuous when we tell ourselves we are learning something valuable about the world – as if mainlining all the tragedies and terrors of humanity 24/7 were some kind of societal obligation. And the awful truth is, it feels good. As Roger McGough wryly observes in this funny little poem, there is a momentary comfort in reading about other lives, more dramatically blighted than our own. It puts our worries into perspective, while releasing just the same quick hit of dopamine that the influencer gets from his selfie, or the gamer from her new in-app purchase. Even the more staid political stories may give us the thrill of superiority, of knowing our side is right and the other wrong – if not (we might tell ourselves) fundamentally malevolent.

These are not noble pleasures. And, as many of us learned during the pandemic, there is a very real psychological toll that comes with remaining constantly abreast of the news. Inviting loss, chaos and fear into our lives as light entertainment may feel rewarding in the short term, but it is a recipe for anxiety and dread in the longer run. So next time you feel a craving for the headlines, perhaps instead you should whip out this little poem, and allow its inherent absurdity to jog you out of the addict's haze.

Survivor
by Roger McGough

Every day,
I think about dying.
About disease, starvation,
violence, terrorism, war,
the end of the world.

It helps
keep my mind off things.

Condition: World-weariness

There are times when this humdrum world, so full of responsibility and routine, can weigh on even the most optimistic of us. Work and home and work again; grey skies and buildings; the predictability of familiar surroundings. Sometimes it can feel that we are not living at all, but merely existing. That is when this rousing little poem comes into its own. Through it, Mary Oliver teaches us that if we want to live life, rather than simply endure it, we must engage our sense of wonder at every opportunity.

The play of light on leaves, the press of a weed through a pavement crack, the rush of a bird in flight (no matter if it's only a pigeon): even in the most prosaic of surroundings, there is always something to spark our wonder, if we can only recognize it. The trick is to take the time to tune into life and into the present moment; to move beyond our world-weariness and see our surroundings through new eyes, even if only for a heartbeat. And then, of course, once we have found the magic, we must spread it. The world, in all its quiet beauty, is made for sharing, for pointing and saying, 'Look. Look!'

Once one begins to be alert to the wonder of the world, there is simply no end of things to be astounded by. The complex web of discoveries, inspirations and relationships that created your toaster; the fundamental physical laws that keep our feet on the ground and our sun in the sky: we are surrounded by miracles, every moment of every day. And yet perhaps the greatest miracle of all is that we do not have to wonder alone. Take a moment, right here, right now, to be astonished. And then, most important of all – find someone to tell about it.

86

Instructions for Living a Life
by Mary Oliver

Instructions for living a life:
Pay attention.
Be astonished.
Tell about it.

Finding Light

Condition: Dissatisfaction with Success

ALSO SUITABLE FOR: *ambition · dissatisfaction with life · need for small pleasures · tunnel vision*

I couldn't begin to count the number of people I've spoken to in my pharmacy who have achieved what many people have only dreamt of, and yet who feel that something essential is still lacking. An indefinable disappointment lurks behind their accomplishments, so that even the pride that they take in them is tarnished; yet to complain seems out of touch at best, and churlish at worst.

When we ask ourselves why we desire success, the answer must always boil down to, 'because I think it will bring happiness'. Why else does anyone do anything, if not for their own happiness or that of the people they care about – whether that be close family, or the entire human race? Worldly achievements are an instrumental good: they are desirable only because of the further good things we believe they can bring.

The error these dissatisfied patients of mine have made is to prioritise their goal over all else – even the happiness they were seeking to begin with. Pleasure can be found in achieving these goals, it's true. But more often, it is found in enjoying life, in nurturing relationships, and in allowing oneself grace and patience. The truth is that a life of small pleasures – of flowers smelled and quiet time shared – is rich in a way that no bank balance can compensate.

The solution here is not necessarily to give up on your goals, but simply to recognize that pleasure is not something to be hoarded away into the future, stored until some later date when everything has come together. Through countless conversations with the rich and powerful, I've learned one simple fact: the less pleasure you can take in the journey, the more likely you'll be disappointed by the destination. It's a question of attitude – and the adjustments needed are available to all of us.

'What sort of life could satisfy the heart'
by Simonides
translated by Christopher Childers

What sort of life could satisfy the heart
    apart from pleasure?
                    What tyrant's treasure
    be worth the having?
                  Pleasure apart,
not even a god's life would be worth living.

Condition: Feeling Past One's Best

ALSO SUITABLE FOR: *disappointment · dissatisfaction with life · loss · setbacks*

Our lives on this earth may not be as long as an apple tree's, but they are still much longer than most of us give them credit for. In the words of another wonderful, but perhaps less cheerful poem, 'Life is very long'. And in a life that contains so many seasons, it is foolish of us to presume that each one will reach the heady heights of the very best of our days. This is a poem that reminds us to recalibrate our expectations, and acknowledge the inevitability of fallow periods in between bountiful harvests.

It's terribly easy when we've had a wonderful experience – be it a friendship, an opportunity, or just a delicious apple – to assume that that should become the norm. But life isn't like that. The reason these things are marvellous is precisely because they are not normal. Life, by necessity, is varied. Like a beautiful orchard, our lives are cast in dappled light and shade. Yes, that means we will sometimes face disappointments – but it also gives us the capacity to be surprised by joy when it blossoms. And who would want it any other way?

The same is true of our own efforts. However talented and brilliant we may be, we will never be producing our best efforts at every possible turn. Of course, like the apple trees in this striking poem, we must always have the optimism – and the sheer joyful determination – to try our best, springing trustingly into action once more at the first signs of thaw. But we must recognize, too, that we do not exist in a vacuum, and we remain at least in part at the mercy of the world's weathers. Some years, the frost returns; some years our hopes are planted in unfertile ground. The key is to forgive ourselves when we don't get the results we'd wanted – and always to keep on trying. Because some years, too, there are apples.

Gather
by Rose McLarney

Some springs, apples bloom too soon.
The trees have grown here for a hundred years, and are
    still quick
to trust that the frost has finished. Some springs,
pink petals turn black. Those summers, the orchards
    are empty
and quiet. No reason for the bees to come.

Other summers, red apples beat hearty in the trees,
    golden apples
glow in sheer skin. Their weight breaks branches,
the ground rolls with apples, and you fall in fruit.

You could say, *I have been foolish*. You could say,
    I have been fooled.
You could say, *Some years, there are apples*.

Condition: Fear of Choice

ALSO SUITABLE FOR: *fear of the unknown • perfectionism • lack of conviction • decision paralysis • false dichotomies • facing dilemmas*

So often when I listen to people's problems, I hear them talking about choice as if were a question of absolutes. Certainly, the right path and the wrong path can strike us as wonderfully easy to differentiate in retrospect. In the moment, however, they are often indistinguishable – and so, as my patients stand at that crossroads, they tear themselves apart trying to divine which is which. How much agony could be prevented if we accepted that sometimes there simply isn't a right answer?

Impossible decisions can be truly agonizing – indeed, the mental anguish of having a choice to make is worse than either option could possibly be. We put upon ourselves an unbearable weight of responsibility, to anticipate every pro and con, to scrutinize the entrails of our lives and become prophets of our own future. There is an answer which will make everything better, we tell ourselves. If only we could be sure of always making the right choice, we would never need to be hurt again.

What if, instead of bashing our heads against this impossibility, we could simply bring ourselves to acknowledge that life is teeming with unknowable complications and repercussions? No choice is simply good or bad, and no decision will ever save us from chance, chaos and the fickleness of Lady Luck. Sometimes we will hurt; sometimes we will be hurt. And sometimes, too, we will have cause to celebrate. But that we can choose at all – that, as this poem puts it, is the little rudder with which we can alter our course through life's rapids, however minutely.

It is all we have. It is ours to use. And as long as we keep choosing – keep living, keep moving – and remain true to what we love and believe, we will have no cause for regret.

Choice
by Lynn Ungar

There isn't a right answer.
There just isn't. The game show
where the bells ring and the points
go up and the confetti falls
because you got the answer
is a lie. The preacher who would assure you
of how to attain salvation
is making it all up. The doctor
who knows just how to fix
what ails you will be sure
of something else tomorrow.
Every choice will
wound someone, heal someone,
build a wall and open a conversation.
Things will always happen
that you can't foresee.
But you have to choose.
It's all we have – that little rudder
that we employ in the midst
of all the eddies and rapids,
the current that pulls us
inexorably toward the sea.
The fact that you are swept along
by the river is no excuse.
Watch where you are going.
Lean in toward what you love.
When in doubt, tell the truth.

Condition: Need for Encouragement

ALSO SUITABLE FOR: *need for affirmation · anxiety · defeatism · lack of support*

First written just over a hundred years ago, this poem has become a fast favourite with the patients who come to my pharmacy. Something about its humour, its light-hearted drive, just makes it all seem so easy.

Sometimes, when we are lost in the mire of our worries and cares, even taking the next step can seem unfathomably hard – let alone embarking on a new challenge. The voices telling us it cannot be done, whether those of the outside world or, more likely, of our own doubt and despair, are simply too deafening – too thick. And yet, as this poem so jauntily reminds us, there needn't be anything intimidating about just having a go.

Even a task which seems overwhelming, impossible, super-human, one that nobody we know of has ever done before, can be broken down to a series of steps; we only have to see what they are. Those steps, in turn, can be broken down further. And then, methodically, cheerfully, with the trace of a grin and a song in our hearts, we can just . . . get started. Perhaps, very occasionally, it will turn out to be impossible. Most of the time, it won't. Either way, and most crucially, we will have done *something*, and probably picked up some new skills along the way. It really is better to have tried and failed than to be left wondering what might have been.

What may surprise you the most, if you take this marvellous poem to heart, is how much easier the challenges of your life turn out to be when you take them a little less gloomily. A heavy heart and a weary sigh can stretch a simple task into days on end of worry. But with a little resolve and a cheerful outlook, a week's problems can be dispensed with before lunch. All it takes is a grin – and getting started.

It Couldn't Be Done
by Edgar Albert Guest

Somebody said that it couldn't be done
    But he with a chuckle replied
That 'maybe it couldn't,' but he would be one
    Who wouldn't say so till he'd tried.
So he buckled right in with the trace of a grin
    On his face. If he worried he hid it.
He started to sing as he tackled the thing
    That couldn't be done, and he did it!

Somebody scoffed: 'Oh, you'll never do that;
    At least no one ever has done it;'
But he took off his coat and he took off his hat
    And the first thing we knew he'd begun it.
With a lift of his chin and a bit of a grin,
    Without any doubting or quiddit,
He started to sing as he tackled the thing
    That couldn't be done, and he did it.

There are thousands to tell you it cannot be done,
    There are thousands to prophesy failure,
There are thousands to point out to you, one by one,
    The dangers that wait to assail you.
But just buckle in with a bit of a grin,
    Just take off your coat and go to it;
Just start in to sing as you tackle the thing
    That 'cannot be done,' and you'll do it.

Condition: Environmental Despair

ALSO SUITABLE FOR: *existential dread · fatalism*

We are all burdened, nowadays, with climate anxiety. For those of us who have reached a later stage of our lives, it's at least easy to tell ourselves that – however grim the news becomes – climate crisis is unlikely to engulf *us*. But where my cohort grew up with the possibility of nuclear winter to darken our hopes, the generations beneath us are faced with the certainty of an environmental, political and humanitarian crisis that is already building steam and, as far as we can tell, is set to worsen dramatically in their lifetimes. In the midst of this existential dread and the very real anxiety it inspires, it can feel utterly impossible to look to the future with any sense of hope or possibility.

That's where this gentle, optimistic verse from Cicely Herbert can come to the rescue. Because although the future is daunting, it is by no means fixed. Everything changes – for the worse, but also for the better. Sometimes, too, the utterly unexpected can emerge from something as simple as a previously unforeseen arrangement of the same old elements. That's partly why the most transformative change, at least within our own lives, is also often the most overlooked. It is a change of perspective.

What this poem so marvellously captures is the difference we can make if we reframe the future and the tasks before us. Perhaps we cannot change everything, cannot save the day in a single grand gesture. But by working towards a better future and finding new ways to fit together the old, well-worn fundamentals of life, in whatever ways we are capable of, however small, we can take some measure of control. Fatalism benefits no one – least of all those born later. As Herbert reminds us, despair can give way to hope. And hope is what we need, if we are to guide this ever-changing world in the right direction.

Everything Changes
by Cicely Herbert

Everything changes. We plant
trees for those born later
but what's happened has happened,
and poisons poured into the seas
cannot be drained out again.

What's happened has happened.
Poisons poured into the seas
cannot be drained out again, but
everything changes. We plant
trees for those born later.

Condition: Hopelessness

ALSO SUITABLE FOR: *angst • despair • facing disaster*

In our human world, ruled as so much of it is by materialism and consumerism, we often feel that the value of a life can be measured by what we've got – or even, sometimes, miserably, by what we haven't got. But one thing that can never be taken away from us is hope. When life is at its darkest, loss is all around us, and we feel utterly bereft, it's natural to fear that things will never get better. As long as we still have hope for the future, however, we can never truly say that we have nothing.

The wonderful thing about hope is that it can flourish in the most barren of places. It asks nothing of us – no struggle, no payment, not even logic. Hope can be felt anywhere, by anyone, in the most unthinkable of situations. Often, the call of hope is strongest in our darkest moments, as if it were nourished rather than depleted by adversity. The singing of that little bird can be heard over the starkest gale, the most deafening tribulation.

When I feel at my most alone, and my most afraid, I try to take a moment to remember this timeless poem, and to hear the song of hope that, as Emily Dickinson so wisely tells us, perches in the soul. Always, if I sit long enough, I can hear its call guiding me through the roaring winds of my turmoil. So next time you feel all is lost, have a listen for that little bird, strong and selfless and deep within. It's been there all along, singing for you, if only you could hear it.

'Hope' is the thing with feathers
by Emily Dickinson

'Hope' is the thing with feathers –
That perches in the soul –
And sings the tune without the words –
And never stops – at all –

And sweetest – in the Gale – is heard –
And sore must be the storm –
That could abash the little Bird
That kept so many warm –

I've heard it in the chillest land –
And on the strangest Sea –
Yet – never – in Extremity,
It asked a crumb – of me.

Condition: Existential Dread

despair at the absurdity of the world

When we find ourselves in the grip of the big existential questions, confronting the sheer absurdity of time, mortality and loss, the temptation can be to rage against the horror of it all. Anger, after all, is the easiest emotion to summon when we do not want to confront our own sadness and fear. The other temptation, just as strong, is denial. If we hide from these realities, we tell ourselves, then they will never find us. If we do not believe in death, or in our own insignificance, then maybe – just maybe – they will not believe in us either.

The truth is that neither of these reactions will ultimately help us to overcome our fear. Instead, we can learn something from this beautiful little poem by Ross Gay, and attempt to greet the great absurdities of life with a sense of gratitude instead. We can learn to say to the world around us, 'Yes, you are terrifying. Yes, you are unfair. Yes, you contain paradoxes and disappointments beyond my imagination. But the very experience of these things, the jarring consciousness at the centre of the human experience, is proof that I am alive in the world.' There is no existence that does not contain these existential woes, because they are at the very core of existence itself.

If we allow it to, the futility and incomprehensibility of life can destroy us. But wouldn't it be better to smile, to laugh, even, and to say, 'Isn't it marvellous that I'm in on the joke?' The world is overwhelmingly vast and mysterious. But we are part of the world. Perhaps we can take solace in the fact that that makes us vast and mysterious, too, and give our thanks for it.

Thank You
by Ross Gay

If you find yourself half naked
and barefoot in the frosty grass, hearing,
again, the earth's great, sonorous moan that says
you are the air of the now and gone, that says
all you love will turn to dust,
and will meet you there, do not
raise your fist. Do not raise
your small voice against it. And do not
take cover. Instead, curl your toes
into the grass, watch the cloud
ascending from your lips. Walk
through the garden's dormant splendor.
Say only, thank you.
Thank you.

Condition: Pessimism

ALSO SUITABLE FOR: *fear for the future • fretfulness • overthinking*

I am often reminded of one of Winnie-the-Pooh's most delightful moments, which comes as he is comforting a frightened Piglet. 'Supposing a tree fell down, Pooh, when we were underneath it?' asks Piglet. Pooh thinks for a moment. 'Supposing it didn't,' he replies. When I am overwhelmed by morbid fear, the doomsaying of newspapers and the terror of the unknown – in other words, when I am being a Piglet – this lovely poem by William Stafford has come to be my very own Winnie-the-Pooh.

Faced with the myriad horrors of the modern world, we can easily live our whole lives in a state of suspended animation, in fear of what might happen tomorrow. Just as easy, though less warned-against, is to pass our days in that state of constant anticipation that longs to see what wonderful thing might happen next – but, rather than running to meet it on its way, only sits and waits. The truth is that we never know what will come, be it wonder or misery. Every moment spent in dread of the future, or in wishing away the present in anticipation of joy to come, is another precious second of our lives gone to waste.

Of course, as Stafford acknowledges, we will always be looking forward – and keeping a look out. Yet we should never lose sight of the bounty of all those things of which we *can* be sure: of the simple pleasures to be found in the morning and evening light, in the unfolding of the here and now. Life is lived in the present. And though there are no grand guarantees in this world, there are still some small certainties. The sun will rise, and crest, and sink again; a new day will come, and it will be ours to savour and reach out towards.

Yes
by William Stafford

It could happen any time, tornado,
earthquake, Armageddon. It could happen.
Or sunshine, love, salvation.

It could, you know. That's why we wake
and look out – no guarantees
in this life.

But some bonuses, like morning,
like right now, like noon,
like evening.

Condition: Need for Spiritual Satisfaction

ALSO SUITABLE FOR: *need for beauty · dissatisfaction with life · need for small pleasures · spiritual hunger · weariness*

Inspired by the Persian poet Saadi and passed hand to hand for over a century, this poem expresses a sentiment whose truth has been known at least since humanity's first cave painting was scrawled on a rocky wall: that an unfed soul is just as great a struggle as an empty stomach. All too often – if certain tabloid headlines and television programmes are to be believed – the instinctual response of the fortunate and the privileged to a poor person spending money on something that actually brings them joy seems to be to lecture, to scold or to sneer. And yet the mere subsistence these sneerers presumably recommend – spartan, dutiful, unleavened by pleasure – almost immediately becomes an overwhelmingly bleak chore. What joy is there in living, if we have no flash of beauty, no moment of wonder to buoy the soul?

By the same token, it can be all too easy to assume that when our bellies are full and our bodies are warm we therefore have no right to feel that anything is lacking in our lives. Any dissatisfaction we feel (so we might tell ourselves) is an expression of our own sense of entitlement, the whining of a spoiled child. As almost everyone's parents and grandparents must have reminded them in their early years, there are places in the world where children are starving. What right have we to feel empty, when we are so literally full?

When we acknowledge the simple truth of these lines, they give us space to understand that our feelings are legitimate. We are indeed starving: not physically, but spiritually. When your subconscious cries out for sustenance, it will do no good to slap it down or shame it for its needs. Instead, give yourself permission to treat it with compassion and grace. Give it the gift of beauty, natural wonder, art or music, or human company. Buy hyacinths to feed the soul.

Hyacinths to Feed the Soul
by James Terry White

If of thy mortal goods thou art bereft,
And from thy slender store two loaves alone to thee are left,
Sell one, and with the dole
Buy hyacinths to feed the soul.

Condition: Second-guessing Happiness

ALSO SUITABLE FOR: *fear of loss • self-sabotage • fear of stability • trust issues*

The great mystery of happiness is that, despite its being the ultimate aim of the vast majority of human endeavour, it is still all but impossible to understand, let alone capture. Why does it refuse to come when we call it, and instead saunter, cat-like, into our lives at the strangest moments? Why does it refuse to stay in the palaces we build to it, and instead make its home in the humblest of surroundings? Why can it never be held longer than it wishes to stay, and never coaxed into following logic or common sense? Truly, the feline inscrutability of happiness is humanity's greatest puzzle.

All of this means that for many of my patients, happiness is a fundamentally uncomfortable condition. They cannot trust it to remain, and therefore they find themselves constantly tensed, ready to dive for cover the moment it begins to recede. It's a funny sort of self-sabotage, making oneself miserable through the anticipation of misery to come. For these patients, I have found that this lovely poem by Naomi Shihab Nye can be transformational. It shows us a new face for happiness, and a new way of coexisting with it.

In this poem, we see happiness not as a goal or an entitlement, but a weather condition. Happiness drifts into our lives like a fog, and cannot be held or bargained with. Instead, Shihab Nye shows us how to bask in happiness, to allow it to flow through and out of us without effort or conflict, brightening the world when it chooses to visit, and leaving unmourned when it departs. The trick is not to ask that happiness remain forever, but instead to trust that it will return, in its own time.

So Much Happiness
by Naomi Shihab Nye

It is difficult to know what to do with so much happiness.
With sadness there is something to rub against,
a wound to tend with lotion and cloth.
When the world falls in around you, you have pieces to pick up,
something to hold in your hands, like ticket stubs or change.

But happiness floats.
It doesn't need you to hold it down.
It doesn't need anything.
Happiness lands on the roof of the next house, singing,
and disappears when it wants to.
You are happy either way.
Even the fact that you once lived in a peaceful tree house
and now live over a quarry of noise and dust
cannot make you unhappy.
Everything has a life of its own,
it too could wake up filled with possibilities
of coffee cake and ripe peaches,
and love even the floor which needs to be swept,
the soiled linens and scratched records . . .

Since there is no place large enough
to contain so much happiness,
you shrug, you raise your hands, and it flows out of you
into everything you touch. You are not responsible.
You take no credit, as the night sky takes no credit
for the moon, but continues to hold it, and share it,
and in that way, be known.

Great Escapes

Condition: Overcome by Sorrow

ALSO SUITABLE FOR: *need for initiative • feelings of powerlessness*

When we are almost engulfed by sorrow, when we feel the waters crashing over our heads and fear they may drown us completely, it may seem to us that we will never reach dry land. In these moments, there is a great temptation to allow ourselves to sink beneath the tumult of the waves to the relative calm of despair. Withdrawing from life, and from the exhausting effort to stay afloat, can seem like a relief.

This poem, by the marvellous Langston Hughes, offers us another solution. If we can find the strength, he tells us, we can take the very sorrow that threatens to drag us beneath the surface, and instead use it to propel us forwards. We can catch the wave instead of being buffeted by it. Sorrow need not be numbing and draining; it can also be a passion, one which can be channelled just as any other passion can be. Its strength and its power to move us, both literally and figuratively, can be exactly the impetus we need to heal ourselves.

When we feel powerless beneath our sorrows, it can be a compounding misery which makes everything else even harder to bear. But if we can galvanize ourselves to *use* our sorrows with purpose, it is astonishing how constructive it can be. Sadness presents us with opportunities to better know ourselves, to rebuild the parts of us that have been damaged with greater intention and purpose. And, above all of this, it is a marvellous motivator for change in our lives. Taking control, making the active choice to use our pain constructively – this is the first step towards transformation. With the help of this little poem, we can propel ourselves out of the gloom of those deep waters, and to the sunny shores beyond.

Island
by Langston Hughes

Wave of sorrow,
Do not drown me now:

I see the island
Still ahead somehow.

I see the island
And its sands are fair:

Wave of sorrow,
Take me there.

Condition: Need for Calm

When patients come into my pharmacy feeling overwhelmed, overhung by dark clouds and jittery with anxiety, it can be difficult for them to imagine what calm would actually feel like. It has been a while since they allowed themselves to feel a moment of peaceful contentment, or managed to lower the volume on their racing thoughts long enough to hear the birdsong outside their own heads. At times like that, what they truly need is a moment of stillness; a moment to feel that the world is fashioned not from futilities, but from possibilities.

I have found that Louise Glück's poem 'The Undertaking' has a wonderful way of providing just such a small oasis in a hectic interior life. Many in the psychological profession these days espouse the benefits of visualization as a technique for lifting people out of their difficulties, giving them a glimpse of the mental state they are aiming towards and empowering them to reach out for it. And what could be a more soothing, more uplifting picture of a better world than this Nobel Prize-winner's vision of light and water, of drifting safely on benevolent waves?

Glück conjures the absolute comfort of rocking on a river, away from strife and towards good fortune. In reading, you might be reminded of the story of the baby Moses, set adrift in a basket down the Nile to escape a massacre, soon to find safety as the adopted son of a princess. Then again, perhaps this will strike you as a journey undertaken much later in life. Either way, the poem reminds us, miracles do happen. The peril will pass. There will be a time when you can breathe deeply again, surrounded by the gentle embrace of the elements, and everywhere you turn will be luck. Picture it; let its calm enter into you. You may find that keys begin to turn, and doors to open.

The Undertaking
by Louise Glück

The darkness lifts, imagine, in your lifetime.
There you are – cased in clean bark you drift
through weaving rushes, fields flooded with cotton.
You are free. The river films with lilies,
shrubs appear, shoots thicken into palm. And now
all fear gives way: the light
looks after you, you feel the waves' goodwill
as arms widen over the water; Love,

the key is turned. Extend yourself –
it is the Nile, the sun is shining,
everywhere you turn is luck.

Condition: Disconnection from Inner Child

It is dismayingly simple, in our frenetic, often urban adult lives, to lose track of the cores of ourselves. We expend so much energy on maintaining our facades, remaining appropriate and professional and closed off, that we simply have none left over to nourish our inner children. Trapped behind our masks, they wither and fade until something utterly essential to our sense of self seems to have been lost. Meanwhile, we chase achievements and acquisitions, the value of which our child-selves would never understand. Thus, self-alienated, alienated even from our sense of wonder, we spend our days chasing enjoyment at the expense of true joy.

When I meet a patient suffering from this malady, I like to prescribe a little holiday from the adult world in the form of this marvellous poem. In it, E. E. Cummings conjures all the childhood magic of the seaside. In an island nation like the Poetry Pharmacy's homeland, the UK, I find it is extremely rare that I meet any patient who does not have deep-seated memories of the freedom and innocence of the beach. The unbounded creativity that can be achieved with bucket and spade; the delightful mystery and horror of a rock pool; the exhilaration of a fierce wave – these are treasured experiences from a time when most of us still encountered the world with an immediacy we might now find startling.

As Cummings so incisively observes, the sea is a place to find ourselves when we are lost. It bears the imprint of our early joy at the enchantments of the natural world, and the wonder of fresh-eyed discovery. When I read this poem, I am transplanted back to a life before deadlines, before any of the trivial adult anxieties that dominate our lives. I find myself – salty, wind-blown, slightly sunburnt, and falling in love all over again with the world around me.

maggie and milly and molly and may
by E. E. Cummings

maggie and milly and molly and may
went down to the beach(to play one day)

and maggie discovered a shell that sang
so sweetly she couldn't remember her troubles,and

milly befriended a stranded star
whose rays five languid fingers were;

and molly was chased by a horrible thing
which raced sideways while blowing bubbles:and

may came home with a smooth round stone
as small as a world and as large as alone.

For whatever we lose(like a you or a me)
it's always ourselves we find in the sea

Condition: Over-indulgence

ALSO SUITABLE FOR: *boredom with plenty • inability to delay gratification • hedonism • need for self-discipline*

In the Western world, we are obsessed with the idea of *having*, sometimes to the exclusion of all other pleasures. The need to possess, to consume, to feast and hoard, has become hardwired into our capitalist society until we cannot conceive of taking joy in *not* having anything. The yearly, quarterly, even monthly fashion cycles; new tech releases with improved specifications that hardly seem to improve our experience; bigger and bigger TVs, fridges, cars. Our lives are governed by our appetites, and those appetites seldom go unfulfilled for long.

It's easy to forget, in such conditions, that there is a reason asceticism has been seen as a path to spiritual fulfilment by cultures and religions across history. Going without sharpens the mind, and helps us to focus more clearly on what it is we truly desire. Fleeting whims and pleasure-seeking urges diminish when we take the time to allow ourselves to experience want for longer than the two minutes it takes to order a takeaway. Learning to find enjoyment in restraint is a skill that we could all use a little more of these days – for reasons environmental as much as psychological.

While for most of us the wine merchant and shopkeeper of this poem by Edna St Vincent Millay may long ago have been replaced by the supermarket, its message couldn't be more timely. Learning to make do with less is not, of course, always a choice; and as we arrive at what sometimes feel like the last days of an era of over-abundance and decadence, it may come to be so for even fewer of us. But if we can learn now to extricate ourselves from the monotony of a full stomach, and to relish the highs and lows of a life without instant gratification, we will find the benefits go far beyond our wallets and our waistbands.

Feast
by Edna St Vincent Millay

I drank at every vine.
  The last was like the first.
I came upon no wine
  So wonderful as thirst.

I gnawed at every root.
  I ate of every plant.
I came upon no fruit
  So wonderful as want.

Feed the grape and bean
  To the vintner and monger;
I will lie down lean
  With my thirst and my hunger.

Condition: Longing for Certainty

ALSO SUITABLE FOR: *discomfort with ambiguity · binary thinking*

In the adventure stories of our childhoods, there was always a seductive certainty. You chose a side, good or evil. You found your true love, and were made complete by them. A single path, ordained by fate, unrolled like a red carpet before your heroic feet. The world, we were led to believe, was a puzzle that would eventually click perfectly into place.

But the truth, as laid out in this astute poem by Louis Mac-Neice, is that nothing is ever that simple. The world is a wonderful mess of light and dark and all the shades in between. Our lives are too short and our minds too limited ever to understand it in its entirety. No revelation will ever change that. This world is governed by such complexity and chaos that to impose a singular worldview, to expect a simple answer, would be utterly naive.

This is unsettling, of course. We have been conditioned to long for the reassurance of knowing that we are doing the right thing, moving in the right direction, choosing the right person. If we look closer, though, there is a consolation in knowing that, as MacNeice tells us, no road is right entirely. There is no simple binary, no ideal life from which we are falling short. Our choices are our own, and that is more important than any possible extrinsic value.

Adulthood is in part a coming to nuance, to the richness of ambiguity. How would we ever truly love without recognizing our partners' shortcomings? And how, without accepting the world's unknowability, would we ever feel wonder and awe? It is the complexities of life that give it its savour, and the acknowledgement of our own limitations that allows us to be dazzled by the world around us. If we did have the certainty for which we long, it might be exhilarating for a moment; but imagine the boredom of a totally straightforward life.

Entirely
by Louis MacNeice

If we could get the hang of it entirely
    It would take too long;
All we know is the splash of words in passing
    And falling twigs of song,
And when we try to eavesdrop on the great
    Presences it is rarely
That by a stroke of luck we can appropriate
    Even a phrase entirely.

If we could find our happiness entirely
    In somebody else's arms
We should not fear the spears of the spring nor the city's
    Yammering fire alarms
But, as it is, the spears each year go through
    Our flesh and almost hourly
Bell or siren banishes the blue
    Eyes of Love entirely.

And if the world were black or white entirely
    And all the charts were plain
Instead of a mad weir of tigerish waters,
    A prism of delight and pain,
We might be surer where we wished to go
    Or again we might be merely
Bored but in brute reality there is no
    Road that is right entirely.

Condition: Perfectionism

ALSO SUITABLE FOR: *striving for the extraordinary • fear of failure • need for kindness • self-recrimination*

A lot of my patients, I've discovered, are deeply scarred by the drive for perfection. Often, this pressure has been with them since their childhoods. The voice of some figure or other, perhaps a parent or a teacher, has taken up long-term residence in their psyche, pointing out every small misstep as if it were evidence of a terrible flaw in their personality. Perfectionism, once it is lodged in us, becomes one of the most pernicious forms of masochism – often invisible, and yet capable of untold damage.

In this direct and persuasive poem, Friar Kilian McDonnell reminds us that perfectionism robs us of the joy of experiencing the world as it is. How can we feel the rapture of art, or nature, or love, if we are constantly playing the critic? Beauty is flawed, almost by its nature. From Marilyn Monroe's mole to the squint of Michelangelo's David, the transcendent and pristine are enhanced and deepened by a flicker of their shadow. If we are constantly on guard against the imperfect, we lose sight of all the ways in which imperfection enriches us, of the mess and glorious complexity that is, after all, the stuff of life. If we can accept, even glorify, this imperfection in the outside world, surely we should be able to extend the same grace to ourselves.

Psychological studies have confirmed that the easiest route to happiness is simply to lower your expectations. Not *all* the way, of course – just until they're no longer making your life miserable. Similarly, the quickest path to better self-esteem is to set reasonable goals for yourself. It isn't easy; it may take time. But the first step is to listen a little bit more critically to your internal monologue. Would we feel comfortable demanding the things we expect from ourselves of someone else? If not, it is time to rethink – and treat ourselves to a bit of kindness.

Perfection, Perfection
by Fr Kilian McDonnell

'I will walk the way of perfection' – Psalm 101:2

I have had it with perfection.
I have packed my bags,
I am out of here.
Gone.

As certain as rain
will make you wet,
perfection will do you
in.

It droppeth not as dew
upon the summer grass
to give liberty and green
joy.

Perfection straineth out
the quality of mercy,
withers rapture at its
birth.

Before the battle is half begun,
cold probity thinks
it can't be won, concedes the
war.

~

I've handed in my notice,
given back my keys,
signed my severance check, I
quit.

Hints I could have taken:
Even the perfect chiseled form of
Michelangelo's radiant David
squints,

the Venus de Milo
has no arms,
the Liberty Bell is
cracked.

Condition: Changing for Others

ALSO SUITABLE FOR: *fear of being unloved • insecurity • low self-esteem*

There are two key mistakes that I often see my patients make in the early stages of a new love. Some think that their relationship will change them, in some predictable way; others, that they can change for their relationship. Both of these beliefs are false, and they cause no end of trouble. It's not that people don't change. When they do, however – and certainly if it's to be at all lasting – it has to be for themselves, not for anybody else. Usually, too, it won't be forced, but has to happen, on some level, organically.

It strikes me as a fundamental truth of relationships that being oneself is always a good idea. When you try to conform to what you believe your partner wants, you are doing them a terrible disservice. First, you are assuming you *know* what they want (and here, you are almost certainly wrong). And, second, you are setting them up for disappointment, because, try as you might, you won't be able to keep up the charade forever. The moment you begin to mischaracterize yourself, you steer the relationship closer to its end.

But the person you are really hurting when you deceive others is yourself. As this beautifully succinct poem reminds us, our self-knowledge, self-belief and self-expression are precious things. Indeed, they are the most attractive qualities any partner can offer. How, after all, can you find the other half who fits you, if you allow nobody to see your true shape? And how can you feel confident in yourself, in all your innumerable quirks and eccentricities, if you iron out every wrinkle to seem more palatable to others? To contort ourselves to fit others' expectations is not merely uncomfortable – it is counter-productive. And if they don't like us as we are – to hell with them. They were never the one for us.

Indian Summer
by Dorothy Parker

In youth, it was a way I had
    To do my best to please,
And change, with every passing lad
    To suit his theories.

But now I know the things I know,
    And do the things I do;
And if you do not like me so,
    To hell, my love, with you!

Condition: Need for Adventure

ALSO SUITABLE FOR: *boredom with the easy life · claustrophobia · restlessness · self-isolation · stagnation*

We spend so much of our lives in pursuit of ease and content-ment that it can be quite a shock to discover that being comfortable is not always a pleasure. Indeed, an over-abundance of comfort often leads to sluggishness, boredom and a sense of malaise. When I meet a patient whose problem is simply being too settled, and too set in their ways, I like to think that this poem acts as a sort of call to adventure. Although the outside world may be frightening and unpredictable, it is also where life truly happens.

The trouble with comfort is that it can be a mask for so many things. For some, it may be the basis of true happiness, the cul-mination of a long journey of discovering what makes them fulfilled and content. But for others, it can be a cover for anxiety, despair or fear, whether of taking a risk or of confronting the outside world. For those in the latter category, their safe little bubbles can be the locus of a kind of life-encompassing agora-phobia. But unless we are willing to push ourselves, to open the door and leave the warm fireside of our self-imposed confine-ment, we will never know what's out there waiting for us.

What I particularly love about this poem is that it makes no pretence of certainty about what comes next. The world outside our circle of safety may indeed be a cold and confus-ing place. Acknowledging that possibility and sitting with it is an important precursor to action. Because once we accept the fear in our bellies and set out anyway – not because we want to, but simply because we *must* – that is when the snowy landscape opens before us, great and terrible and thrilling in all its beauty and potential.

The Call

by Charlotte Mew

From our low seat beside the fire
Where we have dozed and dreamed and watched the glow
Or raked the ashes, stopping so
We scarcely saw the sun or rain
Above, or looked much higher
Than this same quiet red or burned-out fire.
To-night we heard a call,
A rattle on the window-pane,
A voice on the sharp air,
And felt a breath stirring our hair,
A flame within us: Something swift and tall
Swept in and out and that was all.
Was it a bright or a dark angel? Who can know?
It left no mark upon the snow,
But suddenly it snapped the chain
Unbarred, flung wide the door
Which will not shut again;
And so we cannot sit here any more.

We must arise and go:
The world is cold without
And dark and hedged about
With mystery and enmity and doubt,
But we must go
Though yet we do not know
Who called, or what marks we shall leave upon the snow.

Condition: Frustrated Ambition

ALSO SUITABLE FOR: *need for change · unrealized potential · feeling trapped by one's responsibilities*

So often, patients will arrive at my pharmacy bearing the intolerable weight of a dream never realized – or, worse, never attempted. They come to me, slump-shouldered and heavy, and explain why the thing they have always wanted to do is the very one it is truly impossible for them to achieve. They have responsibilities, they tell me, both to others and to themselves. There is no possibility of change; their conscience simply will not allow it. Commitments have bound them to a hated routine, and it is their sacred duty to remain imprisoned within it.

When I see people trapped in this lifelong bind, I like to bring this poem out to suggest another possibility. In it, Yrsa Daley-Ward addresses exactly the sort of ostensibly dutiful thinking that can leave us trapped – and lead us to resent the ones we blame for our stasis. Of course, for those of us with responsibilities to people rather than farm animals, it will never be as simple as selling them. Yet the underlying truth here is that often, when we think we are acting in the interests of those around us, we have neglected to take the most important step of all: simply to ask them. If we did, we might be surprised to receive the answer that those we love do not want to fetter us in misery; they want to encourage us to find joy. Even if not, we might convince them to release us.

Of course, beneath the convenient excuse of duty, you may find other, deeper reasons not to make a change. Fear, dread, lack of self-belief. But the great news is that these all lie within you, and therefore are within your power to change. Allow yourself to be swept up in the sense of possibility that Daley-Ward conjures, and you may begin to feel them slipping away, one by one. There is nothing you cannot change; not even yourself.

from *Mental Health*
by Yrsa Daley-Ward

If you have made it past thirty
celebrate
and if you haven't yet,
rejoice.

Know that there is a time
coming in your life when dirt settles
and the patterns form a picture.

If you dream of the city but you live
in the country
milk the damn cows.
Sell the damn sheep.

Know that they will be wishing you
well
posing for pictures on milk cartons or
running over lush hills to be counted
at the beginning of somebody else's
dream.
See, they never held you back.
It was you, only you.

Condition: Need for Escape

When I talk to my patients about their dreams and fantasies, I am often struck by the way their eyes brighten and their voices quicken. The thought of the lives they wish they had – often starkly different to their day-to-day realities – inspires a sense of relief and excitement that they simply cannot contain. It is in exactly this state of mind that I imagine the young W. B. Yeats composing this marvellous poem, which describes his own fantasy of a perfectly idyllic existence.

When our lives are at their most challenging, their most unyielding, their most utterly tarmacked and grey, it is important to have somewhere to retreat to, even if it is only in our minds. In fact, the more of a fantasy it is – the less a reality we could plausibly realize – the better. That is the joy of these wonderful verses, which seem to ooze peace and serenity like honey from a comb. When I feel myself utterly alienated from nature, unsettled by my frenetic city life and its constant demands and anxieties, I find in this poem a terrific balm: one that brings with it all the joys I hope my ancestors once felt, living at the pace of nature and her gifts, and capable of shaping their environment with their own hands if they so chose.

My father was a workaholic human rights lawyer, always embarking on a new campaign or project, and never feeling that his time was truly his own. He was never able to get away as much as he would have liked to, and sadly his life was cut short before he could have the slow retirement he so deserved. This poem is where he went for solace in the toughest times of his life. Now I carry it with me, too, as a place of inner safety that the outside world cannot touch.

The Lake Isle of Innisfree
by W. B. Yeats

I will arise and go now, and go to Innisfree,
And a small cabin build there, of clay and wattles made;
Nine bean-rows will I have there, a hive for the honey-bee,
And live alone in the bee-loud glade.

And I shall have some peace there, for peace comes
    dropping slow,
Dropping from the veils of the morning to where the
    cricket sings;
There midnight's all a glimmer, and noon a purple glow,
And evening full of the linnet's wings.

I will arise and go now, for always night and day
I hear lake water lapping with low sounds by the shore;
While I stand on the roadway, or on the pavements grey,
I hear it in the deep heart's core.

What are the poems that mean the most to you?

If they're not in this book, William would love to hear about them.

Email him at william@thepoetrypharmacy.com.

*

The Pharmacy is also on Instagram. Follow us @thepoetrypharmacy.

Index of First Lines

Index of Conditions

Acknowledgements

The editors and publisher gratefully acknowledge the following for permission to reprint copyright material:

ELLEN BASS: 'The Thing Is' from *Mules of Love,* copyright © Ellen Bass, 2002. Reprinted by permission of The Permissions Company, LLC on behalf of BOA Editions Ltd., boaeditions.org. JAMES K. BAXTER: 'High Country Weather'. Reproduced by permission. RAYMOND CARVER: 'Late Fragment', copyright © Tess Gallagher, 1989. Reprinted by permission of The Wylie Agency (UK) Limited. WENDY COPE: 'Being Boring' from *If I Don't Know*, Faber & Faber Ltd, 2001. Reprinted by permission of the publisher. E. E. CUMMINGS: 'maggie and millie and molly and may' from *Complete Poems: 1904-1962*, edited by George J. Firmage, copyright © the Trustees for the E. E. Cummings Trust, 1956, 1984, 1991. Reprinted by permission of Liveright Publishing Corporation. YRSA DALEY-WARD: 'Mental Health' excerpt from *Bone*, Penguin Books, 2014 copyright © Yrsa Daley-Ward. Reprinted by permission of Penguin Books Limited. EMILY DICKINSON: 'Hope is the Thing with Feathers' from *The Poems of Emily Dickinson: Reading Edition*, edited by Ralph W. Franklin, Cambridge, Mass.: The Belknap Press of Harvard University Press, copyright © 1998, 1999 by the President and Fellows of Harvard College. Copyright © 1951, 1955, 1979, 1983 by the President and Fellows of Harvard College. MARK DOTY: 'The Embrace' from *Sweet Machine*, copyright © Mark Doty, 1998. Reprinted by permission of HarperCollins Publishers. HELEN DUNMORE: 'My Life's Stem Was Cut' from *Counting Backwards: Poems 1975-2017*, Bloodaxe Books, 2019. Reprinted by permission of Bloodaxe Books, www.bloodaxebooks.com. T. S. ELIOT: 'East Coker' excerpt from *The Complete Poems and Plays*, Faber & Faber, 1969. Reprinted by permission of Faber & Faber Ltd. HELEN FARISH: 'The White Gate' from *Intimates,* Jonathan Cape, copyright © Helen Farish, 2005. Reprinted by permission of The Random House Group Limited. VICKI FEAVER: 'Coat' from *Close Relatives*, Martin Secker & Warburg Ltd, 1981,